A User's Guide to a Healthy Brain

—◊◊◊—

Written By

Norton S. Beckerman

Published By.
Your Brain's Health Center, Inc.
P.O. Box 7736
Arlington, VA 22207
www.ybhc.info

ISBN: 1500286443
ISBN 13: 9781500286446

Dedication

This book is dedicated to my parents who put up with me during the time when little was known about the brain, and to my wife whose help, support and editorial skills made writing this book possible.

Table of Contents

Introduction

I'm a user of a brain, my brain. My brain had been taking a beating over the years. I didn't know it until it was really hurting, and its ability to function was threatened. My ability to function was threatened.

I had accepted bad memory as a result of a severe hit in the head I got when I was young and the viral encephalitis that I had in the late 80's. It wasn't until I was told that my speech problem was due to "…an incurable, but possibly manageable, nervous disorder emanating from my brain…" that I even connected talking with my brain, and I had long since given-up on memory.

Sure, I knew that my memory had something to do with my brain, but I just thought that was the way it was, and that's the way it will be forever. You are capable of doing what you can do and no more, and your brain dictates that capability. Once it's damaged, it's damaged and mine had been damaged. I had to accept who I was and what I could or couldn't do.

I didn't know that the wiring in my brain kept changing based on what I did and didn't do. I didn't know that my brain's ability to function either got better or worse as I aged. It didn't just stand still. That's particularly true of cognitive skills.

I was lucky. Everything came together for me at the right time, and my motivation to learn what was happening to me not only helped to solve my problem, but provided me with an understanding that I had never had before. It was an understanding of how my brain functioned and why. That understanding gave me insight into my cognitive problems and provided me with the information that I needed to solve them.

Up until the late 90's we lived with an incomplete understanding of the brain, but it wasn't just incomplete. It was incorrect causing doctors and neuroscientists studying the brain to look down the wrong roads.

Based on that earlier understanding it was felt that the human brain was pretty much a passive organ that simply absorbed and distributed information to various parts in the body. That led to the conclusion that the human brain was all about the past.

That understanding of the brain changed in the late 90's when neurogenesis in adults was discovered. Learning that the brain is continuously generating new brain cells (neurogenesis), from the day you're born to the day you die, and adapting its structure based on what it knows and doesn't know (neuroplasticity) brought with it the understanding that the human brain is dynamic. It was realized that the human brain is about the future, not the past. True, the human brain maintains a data storehouse about "…what was…", but only as it pertains to what "…will be…". It was clear at this point that the human brain functioned to survive, and to function effectively it must be healthy. We are unique because of our cognitive abilities, and to remain unique we need to maintain our cognitive health. And that's what this book is all about.

Section One – Something About Me

What Happened?

I'm not a medical doctor. I'm a secondary researcher, writer and presenter that has developed a very deep and personal understanding of the brain. I took my brain for granted for a long time. I took it for granted until I really needed it, and it seemed like it was leaving me. Because of my personal experiences I now understand the importance of good cognitive health and our ability to achieve it at all ages, but it wasn't always like that.

I was born into a first generation American family. I was the first child, the first male, and I was the son of the first college graduate in the family. Yes, I was also the son of the first professional in the family.

Expectations for my future were high. I was supposed to be just like him if not smarter. Maybe one day I would even be President, and that's how I was treated. They didn't know back then that anyone that had brains really didn't want to be President.

All was well with me, and going according to plan, assuming, of course, that they had a plan, until I was about 8 years old. Some friends and I were playing keep-away in the back alley, but we didn't have a ball so we were using a brick, a logical thing for an 8 year old to do. The last thing I saw for 24 hours was the smile on my friend Humphrey's face and a full size, red brick coming right at my head.

I didn't remember when I woke up, and I really didn't remember anything else for quite a while. There was a major change though. Now I was considered to be fragile, and the things that I could and couldn't do were limited and closely monitored. To me, the biggest loss was that I couldn't ride a 2 wheel bike like my friends until I was 13 years old. I can't tell you how embarrassing that was.

The incident with the brick not only produced a pair of very frightened and attentive parents, but almost immediately afterwards I started having seizures. That was why they wouldn't let me ride a 2-wheel bike. They first had to be sure that the seizures were under control.

Imagine how my poor brain felt in all of this. First, it takes this terrible hit. That had to do some damage. There was probably some internal bleeding, badly damaged brain cells and cell networks. That had to have affected my cognitive abilities. Then on top of that came the seizures. They do their own damage.

Fortunately, I did reasonably well at school. Went to college, graduate school, got married, raised a family, and ran my own business, but I wasn't a shining star or a professional like my dad, and I never became President. I was just an average person with an average brain doing what I needed to do to move forward in life.

That was who I was, and I never gave my poor, hurting brain much thought during any of this. I'm sure that I treated my pet dog much better than my brain.

My brain was up there perched on my shoulders and resting comfortably in my skull. I was just taking it along with me for the ride. How was I supposed to know that my brain had the ability to rewire itself to accommodate lost cells and cell networks.

When you're young, physically active and constantly learning you're generating a lot of new, experience-dependent cells and creating new, functional cell, networks. The thing is that if I had worked at it, my brain would have generated even more new cells and new functioning cell networks. I didn't know, and no one told me, because apparently+ no one else knew either.

There was one thing. Regardless of whether my brain could generate new brain cells and restructure itself to accommodate them, I never had a good memory after the brick incident. It wasn't particularly bad. It wasn't particularly good. It was OK, but just OK. That made things difficult, but I didn't give it a second thought. After all, I was banged in the head with a very hard brick. What could I expect?

Life went along. My brain and I went right along with it. That is, until the late 80's when I was hospitalized with viral encephalitis; a virus of the brain. They say that viruses like to attack the weak point in the body. I guess, before attacking, the virus evaluated me, and picked my brain as the best point of attack.

My poor brain! It was bad enough that it had been damaged with a brick, and had suffered through seizures, now this viral stuff, and more seizures. They pulled me and my brain through, but it wasn't easy. At this point I didn't even have my just OK memory. It was pretty well shot, and I was living in a fog. I was in that fog at home for 6 months.

Then one day my brain and I were standing in the kitchen, and the fog lifted. Everything around me looked different. I remember that it was a bright sunny day, perfect for such a coming out event. The first thing I did was call my doctor who promptly told me that he knew I wouldn't die. What a terrible response to such a great event. Then I called my wife who was just as excited as my brain and I. There was only one thing though, as time went on it became clear that even though the fog had cleared my memory had not gotten better. In fact, it was worse than ever.

I had little, if any, working memory, and my short term memory was not far behind. You know the kind of working memory I mean. When someone says dial this phone number. The phone is within reaching distance, but I had to write it down. By the way, for those that don't remember, there was a time when people didn't have cell phones with quick dial numbers. They had to rely on those things that were on a stand or mounted on the wall and didn't move around with you.

Now, my brain and I were handicapped, but we didn't let that get us down. We used available technology to supplement our memory. I went out and got spiral notebooks with 3-5 separations, and some really neat mechanical pencils that came 24 to a box. I just started writing everything down that I felt needed remembering. I would date the page, and I tried to keep subject matter separated but that didn't work too well.

More Problems

What you need to know is that I had developed a light weight, high strength composite, and during this time my wife and I were running a manufacturing firm. Not easy to do without memory, but I had my trusty books for reference, and my wife. I don't know what I would have done without her.

Then, in 1996-97 it started. When I spoke there was a definite phlegmy sound about my voice. You know how people say that you're "hoarse". That's how I sounded, but it was gradually getting worse and worse.

I went to the doctor. He started by treating me for allergies. That didn't seem to do anything so he sent me to an otolaryngologist. Now, that was a trip. After sticking this camera up my nose and down my throat he gave me the diagnosis from heaven. The possibilities, he said, could be anything from a sexual disease to cancer, and he proceeded to name off 5 or 6 in-between. To be sure which it was he would have to perform an exploratory operation.

After the operation he decided that he didn't know what was wrong, and sent me to a speech therapist. All that did was cost about $800 and frustrate the poor therapist. With the help of my primary care physician I periodically saw specialists that we thought might be able to help. No luck!

Over time I lost my ability to speak except in a very, high squeaky tone, and that was getting worse. Eventually, it was hard for me to do even that. The consequence was that I tried to speak as little as possible. For me that was a feat, although I think my friends enjoyed it.

I would periodically seek out a doctor that might be helpful. Then in 2002 I was told that I had an incurable, but possibly manageable, nervous disorder emanating from my brain. You talk about scary. My memory was already pretty well shot. I lost my ability to speak, and now they were telling me I had an incurable brain disorder. By the way, I did try to "manage it" with shots to my vocal chords, but that made it worse. It wasn't manageable.

I didn't know much about my brain, but I knew enough to know that memory and complex communication were two primary cognitive skills. What I didn't know is which of my cognitive skills would be next? I have to tell you that I thought about dementia more than just a few times.

My brain and I had lived together since the very beginning. I just couldn't abandon it. It would have been like leaving a good friend who was drowning. So, I did what I always did when I had a problem. I started to read and write down what I thought was important.

Cognitive Health, Memory, and Focus

Everyone knows what cognitive ability is! It's our cognitive ability that makes us who we are. It's our cognitive ability that makes us human. I knew that. But my memory was bad, I was losing my ability to speak, and now I was told that I had an "incurable nervous disorder emanating from my brain". I had to know what was happening to me.

The first thing that I looked up was "cognitive ability" which also showed a reference to "cognitive functioning". I could function cognitively. After all I was a human. It was my cognitive abilities that were being affected, and slowly taken away from me. Eventually, I would stop functioning cognitively in those areas that were declining, maybe in all of them.

That sounds like splitting hairs, but not really. Think of a person batting in a ball game. Anyone that can hold the bat can swing it. They are functioning as a batter, but there are people that can hit the ball more regularly, and harder, than others. Some can even place it where they want it to go. You would say that these people have a greater ability as a batter. We call it skill, but you don't refer to your ability to perform a cognitive function as a skill. You function cognitively, and you have certain cognitive abilities.

Now that I knew what functioning cognitively meant I could develop kind-of a chart in my head that listed them, and rate myself on each. I got very low marks on memory, and verbal communication which I had expected, but I got some low marks on other things as well, like learning, reasoning and problem solving, that I hadn't expected. I guess you could say that it was enlightening, but it was actually scary, and depressing. I was going downhill mentally.

I should tell you up front that it turns out your brain is responsive to what you do and what you don't do. It determines what you can and can't do as well as what you will and won't do. We'll get into all that later on but my brain and its cognitive abilities were definitely affecting what I would and wouldn't do.

I had to find out what was happening, and if there was anything that I could do to stop it. I never really expected to improve my cognitive abilities. I just wanted to get back to where I was and hold onto them.

I not only regained my cognitive abilities I improved them. Today I have an excellent memory, probably a better memory than I've ever had. I speak clearly. I'm constantly learning and doing new things. I'm mentally sharp, and much more capable of functioning cognitively than when I was younger.

It turns out that "memory" and "focus" are key to understanding cognitive functioning and cognitive ability. Since that's where I was headed, knowing the role that they played in maintaining or losing cognitive ability was a bonus. So, let's start where I started.

THE COGNITIVE PERSON
Cognitive Functioning is..."The ability to obtain, recall, use and relate knowledge (information), thought, experience and learning..."

Cognitive functioning refers to a wide range of capabilities; reasoning, learning, processing visual, auditory, smell, taste and tactile information, understanding, problem solving, being able to relate one piece of information to another, thought, perception, language, complex communication, creativity, and the conveying of thought to another person or translating thought into an external object whether it be an artwork, an artifact, a written paper or a computer.

Cognitive Abilities refer to the degree to which you can do each of these things. You have all of the cognitive functions, but how well can you do each? When you answer that question you describe your cognitive ability, and give meaning to your cognitive functioning. Understanding cognitive functioning and your cognitive abilities tells you who you are.

Memory and Focus – Memory is the key to functioning cognitively. Memory is the key to learning. It's your memory that allows you to relate, interpret, and prioritize bits of stored or newly received information. It's how much, and how accurately, you can remember that determines your cognitive abilities. Your brain shouldn't have any difficulties remembering what's going on internally, and responding. It's the external information that your brain is receiving, or not receiving, from its sensors that presents the problem. That brings us to "focus".

Your ability to focus on the information that your brain is receiving from external sources establishes the accuracy and comprehensiveness of your memories. The internal health of your brain, its ability to function mechanically, will affect both your focus and your memory. Go back to the batter. If you have a person that is outstanding at hitting the ball, but that person has a sore wrist or arm he or she won't perform as well. The same is true of your brain. If those things in your brain that allow you to function effectively are hurting or damaged then you won't perform as well either. You want to keep your brain healthy so that it performs well.

MEMORY
Your brain receives images from your eyes, sounds from your ears, smells from your nose, tastes from your tongue, and sensations from what you touch and feel. To the brain that's all information. The brain remembers, or attempts to remember, information that it has received and is storing based on the priority that it has attached to it. Bits of information that are related are stored in

relative proximity to each other. There are pathways that connect them. Receiving the same information from more than one source expands the pathways and makes the memory stronger. The relationship between bits of memory also becomes stronger.

The brain establishes priority based on information previously received and stored. Information that has little or no priority is located deep in the brain's data storehouse or is discarded.

If your brain doesn't have the physical capability to remember the information that it is receiving you won't be able to make a memory and you won't be able to relate bits of memory to each other. That's why the health of your brain is so important.

Now we know that your brain creates memories based on the information it receives, interprets, prioritizes and stores. It can't make memories if it's not receiving information, and it can't make accurate memories if it's not receiving accurate information. That sounds silly, but it will eventually become clear as to why that's important.

The memories that the brain creates are related to other memories, and maintained as information or, if you prefer, data that can be retrieved when needed. Your cognitive abilities are contingent upon memories, data, and information that your brain has stored with relevance and priority. If your cognitive ability in any area is declining, as was happening to me, you could lose your entire ability to function cognitively in that area. I was determined not to let that happen to me. I'm happy to report that it didn't.

YOUR REALITY
Using the memories that it has stored your brain creates your reality. Yes, your reality. Think about it. Your brain is accumulating, evaluating and prioritizing information. It is relating that information to the information that it already has and interpreting it based on an understanding of information previously received and interpreted. That describes what your brain knows. It's what you know.

Your brain only knows what it knows. It only knows what it has learned. It doesn't know any more. What your brain knows is what determines your reality.

A child touching a hot fire is a perfect example. Prior to touching the fire the child did not know that the fire was hot, and that it would burn if touched. The fact that fire was dangerous was not part of the child's reality. They had not previously received the information in such a way that it was meaningful and could be prioritized. Then the child touches the fire. It's hot. It hurts. It has now received, interpreted and prioritized new information. That information was added to the child's data bank. In the future that child will see fire as a painful threat. The fact that fire is dangerous has now become part of the child's reality.

THE BRAIN'S DATA WAREHOUSE
The information that your brain receives and converts into memories is stored at points of connection, called synapse. Your brain produces new points of connection, or synapse, based on the new information you process. Those synapse become a data warehouse for the brain. It then retains a map of where those synapse are located and the memories stored there which, by the way, can be fragmented and spread all over the brain. The strength and ease of retrieval of those memories is established by the brain based on their frequency of use and ascribed importance.

When new information is received by the brain it has to be processed and possibly stored. Your brain uses new, experience dependent cells, cell networks and connections between cells to handle and process this new information. When this takes place your brain is establishing new connections between cells.

Functioning brain cells must draw blood to stay alive. A memory's frequency of use will not only determine where it's stored, but how much blood it will draw. This fact is extremely important in determining how your brain will function.

FOCUS

Focus is all about receiving information completely and accurately so that when it's transmitted back to the brain there will be an accurate and complete interpretation of the sound, noise, image, smell, taste, etc.. As we age, focus becomes increasingly difficult. Some of that loss of focus is physical, some due to life content, and some due to preoccupation with other things. It's like when I do something that has a bad result. My wife might say, "...I told you what would happen if you did that ... You weren't listening." Was it that I wasn't listening or just unable to focus on what was being said. That's a fine line. I don't have focus problems any longer, but I've learned to say "... Yes, I'm sure you did ... I just wasn't listening..." Unfortunately, people with focus problems will say the same thing.

Since the information stored by your brain is what produces your memories, inaccurate, incomplete or a distorted understanding of information received will call your memory into question. That makes focus the key element in producing accurate memories, and a key element in shaping your reality. Fortunately, there are things that can be done as we age to improve, and even enhance our ability to focus. Increasing your ability to focus will help your memory, and probably your relationship with your wife or partner.

Let's go a little further. Your ability to focus is dependent on two different things; the health of your sensory devices and your brain's ability to produce certain neurotransmitters, primarily dopamine.

The health of the sensory devices that produce sight, hearing, smell, taste, touch and feel is critical to the receipt of accurate information from your surroundings. The health of these sensory devices and their capability to transmit information accurately will normally decrease with age. Your vision and hearing are the two senses that generate the most external information. That makes them important to the effective functioning of your brain.

Secondly, the brain produces two neurotransmitters that are essential to focus, dopamine and norepinephrine. Norepinephrine is actually derived from your production of dopamine. There's an easy way to look at focus using these two neurotransmitters. Dopamine is the neurotransmitter that directs your attention to a specific sight, sound, smell, taste, touch or feel. It's the dopamine response that alerts you. Norepinephrine blocks out the surrounding information so that you are focusing on the information that's being received, and that's important. In that way your brain can make an accurate memory. You could say that the dopamine you generate is out in front taking in what's important, while the norepinephrine is holding back the crowd.

Historically it seems that as we get older dopamine production decreases. The crowd is making background noise, and keeps getting closer to what we want to pay attention to. That decreases our ability to focus, to make memories, and to learn. You know the saying "Old dogs can't learn new tricks" implying that age alone is the cause, but that's not true. You can increase your production of dopamine and norepinephrine at any age, while sharpening your ability to focus.

Dopamine is a neurotransmitter that is responsive to an increase or decrease in physical exercise or activity, diet, the learning of new things, and outlook. With positive events and outlook dopamine production increases. With negative events, and outlook it decreases.

I Could Do It!

Once I understood cognitive functioning, and the role that memory and focus played in maintaining and building them I was able to develop some direction to my efforts. Interestingly, at this point I just assumed that my memory was going to be what my memory was, and I would have to live with it. I didn't know how wrong I was.

The first book that I read about the brain had to do with the science of memory. It wasn't really a book, book. It was actually a compilation of papers, talks, and round-table discussions that were presented at a conference by leaders in the field.

Since I didn't have very much of a memory, I started to write. First, I began underlining with the intention of going back over the material, then making asterisks with subject notations, then writing questions in the margins, then writing challenges to statements. I did this in the margins of a page as well as in the front and back fly leafs.

Between a good medical dictionary, my computer, my local library, and good book stores I was able to get through it. I even understood it. When I finished there were notes, questions and writing everywhere. As I look back on it I was fortunate to have started where I did.

There were four things that became very clear from my first reading about the brain. First, these people had developed a language of their own and it was their primary form of communication. This esoteric language was intended to facilitate communication between professionals, but its effect was to shut others out. If I was going to understand what they were talking about, and put it to use, I had to understand the language.

Secondly, there was an incredible amount of new information that was coming forth. The newly evolving technology was providing information about the adult human brain that had not been seen before.

Third, there were all kinds of supporting and contradictory theories about what this new information meant, and how it should be applied. The experts were competing in an effort to understand what was being offered to them. That helped to level the playing field somewhat. I was getting in on the ground floor.

Finally, no one talked about or discussed the function of the brain, and how memory and speech were related to it. It was all about pieces and parts in the brain, like engrams, and how this new information affected them. Engrams, by the way, are bits of information that are stored in the brain, and retrieved through the process of memory and recall.

By the time I got to this point I had associated memory with the functioning brain, but I looked at the act of speaking as a physical function. What would my brain have to do with it? The doctors said it did, but they couldn't tell me what, and apparently neither could the folks at this conference. But I did get quite a bit from my first reading.

I began to understand that the brain was a mystery that neuroscientists wanted to unlock and that there were contradictory opinions about what all of this new information coming forth meant. That conference provided me with the knowledge, understanding and motivation to continue reading, and read I did. I read and learned everything I could about the brain and cognitive function. And I'm still studying and learning today.

Learning How To Speak

At some point in my studies I concluded that I had taught myself how not to speak. In actuality, I had unknowingly rewired my brain so that I couldn't speak. If that was the case then I had to learn how to speak all over again, but not as a child, as an adult. I had to learn a new skill, and I had to teach it to myself. Based on what I had read I approached it as if I was learning to play a musical instrument.

My vocal chords were the instrument. I had to learn how to play them. Power Point held my music and recorded the sounds I made. The slides that it contained were my music book, and my ear phones allowed me to hear the music I was making.

When I began, the text on the slides was limited to no more than a short sentence. As I progressed, the text on the slides got longer and more complex. Breathing exercises helped to prepare the instrument for play, and the brain to expel air in a coordinated manner. That allowed me to make a controlled, or shaped, sound.

I discarded some breathing exercises as not being useful. Some I retained, and some I modified. My headset with its microphone gave me a platform on which to play the instrument, and a way to hear what had been played. I was providing my brain with new information. That new information required an action, speaking. At first, that action was limited and rough, but as time went on the action that I was capable of was expanded and refined.

I would practice 5 mornings a week for about 3 hours each morning. I was definitely making progress. I continued. It took me about a year and a half before I cut the 5 mornings of practice back to 4 mornings, then to 3 mornings, and eventually, to 1 morning. Then I decided I didn't need to practice at all. I had re-trained my brain. I had learned how to play my vocal chords so that I could speak clearly, in a good tone, and with confidence. I could go back out in the world. It seemed that the incurable nervous disorder that was emanating from my brain was curable after all.

SUDOKU and OTHER THINGS

Before we go any further I have to tell you that during all of this time I wasn't just sitting around reading my "brain books" and taking notes. I learned html code which is the code used to write web sites. I designed, wrote material, and put up a site which had nothing to do with the brain. I reacquainted myself with the piano, and my wife introduced me to Sudoku.

Sudoku was just becoming popular. Diane recognized it as a puzzle that required logic and reasoning, two things she always thought I could improve on. Truth is she just didn't understand my logic and way of reasoning.

She and I immediately went out and bought a bunch of Sudoku books. I thought that they would help explain the puzzle, and how to solve it. They were all pretty much alike. Fortunately, their approach confused me. I say fortunately because it forced me to develop my own approach which was to try and do the puzzles in my head, and not write a character in a space until I could actually solve for that space. In retrospect, it turned out to be a great idea.

I thought that I was just engaging myself as a way to pass time. I didn't realize that the approach that I had taken to working the puzzle had forced me to increase focus, and to stimulate memory and reasoning. These were the things that I needed to be doing even if I didn't know it at the time. I eventually called this approach "Mind Sudoku". I guess I should call it "Brain Sudoku" because, with all of the other things I was doing, it really helped to sharpen my cognitive abilities.

Section Two – A Look at the Brain

The Rules that Guide the Functioning

of the Brain

Nothing I did was high tech. It just took a lot of plodding and persistence.

I learned the language, and got things sorted out. At least, I thought that I had, but the onslaught of information that I was trying to absorb was overwhelming.

I wasn't just trying to absorb information directly related to the brain. I was looking for information that affected the functioning of the brain. That information seemed to come from all different directions. With the onslaught of information that I was uncovering it was difficult to sort it out so that I could understand how it all related.

I felt like I was putting together a super-large jigsaw puzzle without having a picture to guide me. Sometimes the pieces fit together, but most of the time it was just a lot of information that I was trying to apply to that thing sitting on my shoulders, my brain, and it wasn't telling me what I needed to know. I decided to take my brain off of my shoulders and start looking at it as an entity. I objectified it. I viewed my brain as if it were another person, an unhealthy person that I had to nurse back to health.

Things started to look different. Initially I was collecting information that seemed to have an isolated role, and in some cases I wasn't sure exactly what that role was. Once I took my brain off my shoulders and looked at it as an entity I realized that these apparently isolated bits of information had to relate to each other in some way. There had to be rules of association.

That sounds way out there, but it wasn't. If there were rules that related the different pieces of information that I was receiving to each other than the picture to my jigsaw puzzle would start to take shape and become clear. I needed to study new information, but I had to go back and look at the information that I had already been through. This time I needed to know how that information related to the other bits of information.

As it turned out there were rules of association. They didn't just fall out. It took time and understanding. There were 6 rules that I was able to identify fairly quickly based on what I already knew. The first rule jumped out at me almost immediately, but I didn't really understand its full meaning until later on down the road.

Rule 1
All living organisms strive to survive … the brain is a living organism therefore the brain must survive.

Everything else is related to that first rule, the rule of "*survival*". I know that it's silly to be talking about survival in our day and age, but the need to survive was the earliest motivation driving the actions of the brain, and it's the motivation that drives the actions of the brain today. If you think about it there were 4 things that drove the earliest human: 1) the need for water, 2) the need for food, 3) the need to avoid predators, and 4) the need for shelter. Those are the same things that drive us today albeit in a much more complex, and frequently obscured, way.

Rule 2
Nothing that the brain does is serendipitous or without purpose. Everything the brain does when initiating an action has a "purpose". That purpose is "survival".

Rule 3
The brain controls the actions of everything contained in, and extending, from it."

Rule 4

The brain only knows what it has learned. The brain only knows what it knows. The actions taken by the brain are the result of what it knows.

Rule 5

The brain equates reward with survival. All actions that are rewarded help to ensure survival and should be repeated. Actions that do not provide reward should be avoided.

Rule 6

The internal and external elements that the brain uses grow, or change, as the survival requirements of the brain grow, or change. The brain establishes its survival requirements based on what it knows. (This rule leads to the brain's toolbox, the Brain-body System.)

As I saw it those first 6 rules provided structure, guidance and direction to the way that the brain functioned. It was easy to sum it up. The way in which the brain functions is guided by its:

    A. need for *Survival,*

    B. actions taken with *Purpose of survival,*

    C. *receiving a Reward* for correct actions

The difference that uncovering those first six rules made was unbelievable. I used them to understand the information that I was receiving. What was previously unruly and overwhelming was making sense. The information seemed to organize itself, and as it did it was drawing a picture. The elements of that picture came from mainstream science. All I was doing was assembling the information and drawing the picture so that it made sense to me.

MY BRAIN and ITS TOOLBOX

Looking at these rules the first thing that became clear was that

> *My brain is not an organ in my body...*
> *My body is an extension of my brain.*

My body is comprised of the tools that my brain needs to survive. My brain is the control and my body is its tool box. That makes it a Brain-body System. Wow! That was a lot to absorb. It was time to take a closer look at that thing that I had taken down off my shoulders. That may not be the way that they teach neuroscience students about the brain, but it was how I understood it, and it was quite useful. My next step was to look at the brain as a whole.

The Functioning Brain

After all of my reading about the human brain with all of its complexities, it's myriad of pieces and parts, and this does that and that does this, I decided to simplify it. I divided the Functioning Brain into 3 parts; The Primary Brain - the Boss, and its two assistants, the Emotional sub-Brain, the Bodyguard, and the Logical Executive sub-brain, the Advisor.

Each of the sub-brains is part of an overall system within the Functioning Brain, but each of these sub-brains is a system unto itself, comprised of its own pieces, parts and connections distributed throughout the brain. Each of the sub-brains has its own set of tools and draws blood to support the functioning of those tools. Each of the sub-brains uses its tools to help ensure the safety and survival of the Primary Brain.

THE PRIMARY BRAIN – THE BOSS
The Primary Brain is that portion of the Functioning Brain that neuroscientists call the Primitive Brain. I don't know why. It's still with us, and it's still controlling what we do, when we do it, how we do it, and why we did it. The Primary Brain is the Boss. Everything else, internal and external to it, is intended to assist in ensuring its survival.

THE EMOTIONAL SUB-BRAIN – THE BODYGUARD
The Emotional Sub-brain came along next. Its job is to scour the environment for threats. The Emotional Sub-brain is the Primary Brain's body-guard. The Emotional Sub-brain does not reason or solve problems. Its receipt of information is literal, and its communication back to the Primary Brain is in the simplistic terms of safety, fight or flight.

THE LOGICAL EXECUTIVE SUB-BRAIN – THE ADVISOR
The Logical Executive Sub-brain came along later, and is much more complex than the Emotional Sub-brain. I guess you could

call it "The Advisor". Like the Emotional Sub-brain, the Logical Executive Sub-brain has the responsibility of protecting the Primary Brain. Its tools for doing so are its cognitive abilities. That makes its communication to the Primary Brain much more complex than that of the Emotional Sub-brain. It also means that it uses a lot more blood.

Everything that the Logical Executive Sub-brain interprets and concludes has to go through the Emotional Sub-brain before it is communicated to the Primary Brain. However, there are times when circumstances require the two sub-brains to communicate with each other, and work out their message to the Primary Brain. The two sub-brains can be very friendly or antagonistic depending on circumstances.

My interest was the Logical Executive Sub-brain. After all, that's where it seemed that my problems existed. It's my Logical Executive Sub-brain that houses and uses cognitive tools. It's my Logical Executive Sub-brain that made me who I was. It was my Logical Executive Sub-brain that was going to determine who I will become.

As my understanding of my Logical Executive Sub-brain increased my anxieties about my future decreased. I realized that, even though my brain was hurting, there were things that I could do to restore it to good health. That meant that I could not only stop the decline of my cognitive abilities I could get them back. I didn't expect to be able to expand them, but that's what happened.

I thought I was pretty slick when I got to this point. I didn't realize that I had just gotten to the starting line. You really can't understand the brain, how it functions, and what you need to do to make sure it stays in good shape until you understand the physical laws that govern the growth and death of the brains internal structure, and their implications. I'm referring to neurogenesis and neuroplasticity.

The Laws that Govern the Internal
Structure of the Brain

Until the late 90's it was universally agreed that genetics established a structure that determined what your brain was capable of doing and not doing. It was thought that your brain was what it was, that neither you nor your brain had much say in the matter.

There is no question that genetics are an important resource for the ever-learning child, but genetics are only a starting point. By the time you're a mature adult they probably have little bearing on your mental capabilities thanks once again to the dynamic duo neurogenesis and neuroplasticity.

Neurogenesis and neuroplasticity are both physical laws, and physical tools that govern the structure and composition of the brain. Its neurogenesis and neuroplasticity that are responsible for the continuous rewiring of your brain. They're laws because they operate within your Functioning Brain from birth to death regardless of your age, and you can't turn them off. They are tools because they're used by your brain to help ensure its survival. Unfortunately, neuroplasticity can prove to be a strength, or a weakness, depending on how it's used.

It was my understanding of neuroplasticity and neurogenesis that brought me to the conclusion that I had taught myself how not to speak. We normally think of teaching and learning as being positive and as something that we want to do. But any action that's engaged in repetitively will cause your brain to rewire itself, and that could be good or bad.

I concluded that based on how I was using my voice over the years I had actually taught myself how not to speak, and as a result of the law of neuroplasticity my brain had rewired itself to accommodate what I had learned. If my brain accommodated my learning "how not to speak" it was a small jump to conclude that I could learn "how to speak".

It was neuroplasticity that had taken away my ability to speak. (the law) But it was that same dynamic duo that could give me the opportunity to learn how to speak once again. All I had to do was figure out how to use them (the tool). That's when things became a little dicey.

When you're a small child, speaking comes as a result of genetics, interaction with others, a gradual training of the vocal chords, and breathing. Your brain is hearing, learning and using, hearing, learning and using. To speak it is essential that breathing is coordinated with pronunciation, but the small child doesn't have to think about that.

Genetics should allow the coordination of breathing and pronunciation to come naturally to a child, but I was no longer a child. I was an adult that had learned "how not to speak". I had to learn "how to speak" as an adult. That required that I provide my brain with new information that it could act on, and I had to convince it that "speaking" was of top priority.

I didn't have a roadmap to follow, and I didn't have a reference book to go to so I could see if what I did was correct. I didn't sit around all day saying "Ah-hah!" now I'm going to learn just how I can use neurogenesis and neuroplasticity to talk again. They were new to everyone, particularly me.

Neurogenesis and neuroplasticity are physical laws. The only guidelines you have in learning how to use them is your understanding of what they do, knowing what you want to do, and coming up with some type of plan to get you there. Then, of course, it's repetition and persistence. It's a learning process. It's the same learning process that an athlete or a pianist goes through to perfect his or her skill. For that matter it's the same learning process that anyone goes through that wants to perfect a skill. It's the same process that anyone goes through if they want to learn something.

I wanted to learn how to speak. I had to feed my brain information that it would respond to, but I had to feed it the correct information in the correct way. The only thing that I could think of to do was to try and read things out loud. I knew that breathing was involved because of my trips to the speech therapist, but at this point I didn't know how it was involved or how to use breath to regain my speech.

Neurogenesis and neuroplasticity are the laws that I had to depend on. They guide the physical functioning of the brain. Your brain is your control center. Your brain controls everything but neurogenesis and neuroplasticity. Neurogenesis and neuroplasticity are controlled by what you do or don't do.

Neurogenesis and neuroplasticity exist just like tissue exists. They're there waiting to receive information. How they function within the brain depends on the information that it's receiving and how it's being received. The information that the brain receives depends on what you do or don't do.

If what you are doing produces new information it has to be processed. Processing means new cells and new or larger cellular networks. There has to be space for these new cells and cellular networks. That's when neuroplasticity steps in. Neuroplasticity makes the space, creates connections and lays down new pathways for communication. That allows blood to be drawn to the area.

If there is no new information to process new cells or cellular networks aren't needed. No additional space or pathways are necessary and neuroplasticity doesn't have a roll to play. Not yet anyway.

Neurogenesis and neuroplasticity function based on what the brain knows and what it's learning. Without neurogenesis and neuroplasticity we would be stuck in the moment, unable to learn or accommodate new things or new information. That suggests that neurogenesis and neuroplasticity have a significant influence on our cognitive skills.

It's hard to separate neurogenesis and neuroplasticity, since for the most part, they operate together. However, each has components that operate independently. Neurogenesis seems to be the least complicated so I'm going to start there.

NEUROGENSIS
The saying "You can't teach an old dog new tricks" mentioned earlier refers to our ability to learn new things when we got older. For generations it was believed that the brain you had when you were born developed until you were about 20, but you were done after that. Your brain was what it was, and there wasn't much you could do about it. As it turns out that wasn't true.

Approximately 30 years ago it was discovered that you could teach adult songbirds new songs. The ability to learn new songs showed that the songbird was able to create, process, and use new cells. These new cells were responsible for the bird's retention of the new songs. Teaching the bird new songs was allowing them to make new memories. That implied the existence of a relatively complicated, functioning network of new cells. It also meant that the circulatory system in the bird's brain had to support these new cells and cell networks.

At the time, nothing much was made of the discovery. It was not applied to humans, and it certainly wasn't applied to adult humans. After all, it was well known that the adult human brain couldn't grow new brain cells. Then, in the late 90's it was discovered that not only did adult humans grow new brain cells, but the human brain generated new brain cells from birth to death.

Assisting in the growth of new brain cells are chemicals that the brain generates. Those chemicals are referred to as "Brain Derived Neuronal (Growth) Factors", or "BDN(G)F" for short. Even though your brain will generate new brain cells throughout your life the rate at which those cells are produced is pretty much determined by two things; the amount of BDNGF that is produced, and the new information being received that needs processing. That suggests that the rate at which your brain produces new cells is, to a large extent, determined by what you do or don't do.

The Law of Neurogenesis would create a serious problem if it wasn't for the Law of Neuroplasticity. Without Neuroplasticity your brain would just keep making, and making, and making, brain cells until your skull exploded. The relationship of the two laws told me that there are some rules. First, brain cells don't just hang around forever. They have to be used and become active within a relatively short period of time. If they're not used they simply die off. New brain cells are experience dependent and are only used to process new information.

Newly activated cells will have to draw blood if they are to survive. To draw blood the newly activated cells have to belong to a new or existing cellular network. To complete the cycle, brain cells can only belong to a new cellular network if they provide new information, and they can only belong to an existing cellular network if they strengthen the function of that cellular network.

New information is required to strengthen the function of an existing cellular network. When new brain cells are activated and retained they have to go somewhere. Space has to be made to fit them in. New pathways and connections for signaling have to be laid down. Blood has to have a way of getting to the new cell. That's where neuroplasticity comes in.

NEUROPLASTICITY

When I was explaining neurogenesis I said that for generations it was believed that the brain you had when you were born developed until you were in your early 20's, but you were done after that. Your brain was what it was, and there wasn't much you could do about it. The hosting and use of new brain cells was not an issue. It wasn't possible. We believed that connections, signaling and the use of resources (blood) were fixed after a certain age.

If you carry that thought out you realize that we believed that humans beyond their early 20's couldn't learn new things. We believed that once you're an older adult your brain is what it is. That was obviously the belief that prompted the saying "Old dogs can't learn new tricks." By adopting that saying, which was quite popular, we were expressing our belief that the human brain was all about the past. How disillusioning is that, particularly since we're living longer and longer. We would be doomed to doing less and less of the same old things over and over again. But, we're not.

The discovery of neuroplasticity revealed that our brain is continuously reorganizing its pathways, connections and structure to accommodate new cells (neurons) as well as dead and dying cells (neurons). The law of neuroplasticity makes this accommodation by laying down new pathways and closing off others based on what we do or don't do. But this isn't done randomly.

Neuroplasticity has two objectives when laying down and closing off pathways and rewiring connections. The first objective is to strengthen communications, or signaling, between cells and cell networks. The second is to conserve a very valuable resource. In the case of the brain that resource is blood.

When I first started learning about neurogenesis and neuroplasticity it was clear that these two things represented a remarkable advance in brain science. I heard lectures and read studies that related neurogenesis and neuroplasticity to learning, practicing and repetition. I understood that somehow I had learned "…how not to speak…" and I had to relearn "…how to speak…". I understood all of that. But, I didn't understand the impact that neurogenesis and neuroplasticity had on my life in general. I didn't understand what they actually meant.

It wasn't until I was trying to explain these two physical laws to others that I actually realized there importance. This dynamic duo was constantly with me monitoring what I did and didn't do, and adjusting the connections in my brain accordingly, primarily in my Logical Executive Sub-brain. Neurogenesis was giving me the opportunity to grow while neuroplasticity was altering the structure that controlled my cognitive abilities. All of this was being done based on what I was and wasn't doing.

Because of neuroplasticity, learning affects the brain in two different ways. When receiving new information related to already existing connections the connections between neurons are strengthened. A good example would be learning a new piece of music by memory on an instrument that you already know how to play.

If the information being received is brand new the brain will form new connections, and new functional networks, between cells. A good example of that would be learning how to play a musical instrument for the first time.

Initially, neuroplasticity was the brain's internal survival mechanism. Your brain still has that mechanism and the drive to use it. Your brain is continuously adapting to new environments, seeking ways to avoid predators, trying to locate potable water, obtain nutrition, and find shelter. It does all of these things so that it can stay safe and survive. In order to do all of these things your brain is constantly looking for new information.

I understood all of that intellectually, but it took quite a while before I actually understood what it meant to me. Because of neurogenesis and neuroplasticity the brain, my brain, your brain, isn't about what was. Our brains are not about the past. Our brains, and the way that they function, are about what needs to happen to keep us safe in the future. That sounds great, but as far as we are concerned it gives neuroplasticity an upside and a downside.

Think about it. The law of neuroplasticity causes the internal structure of the brain to be continually changing based on what we do or don't do. That change focuses on the Logical Executive Sub-brain, your Advisor, and the sub-brain responsible for your cognitive skills. Those cognitive skills include memory, learning, reasoning, problem solving and complex communication.

Your brain is always looking for new information to process. As long as your brain is receiving and processing new information your Logical Executive Sub-brain with its cognitive skills is needed by the Primary Brain to ensure its safety. Safety and survival go hand in hand. The law of neuroplasticity supports the brain's need to survive by making sure that the communications between cells (neurons) is quick and effective. It also supports the brain's need to survive by making sure that the resources available to the brain, in this case blood, are being used efficiently.

You can be a child, an adolescent, a young adult, a middle-aged or senior adult. Neuroplasticity is functioning to satisfy its two responsibilities, effective communication and resource conservation. Neuroplasticity does this based on what you do or don't do, at all ages. Not just when you're an older adult.

Now comes the bad part. The laws of neurogenesis and neuroplasticity tell us that our brain is continuously changing, and that change is based on what we do or don't do, regardless of age.

We, as a society, have focused on children and young adults as the only ones that need to process new information and learn new things. If we're responsible caregivers we help them accomplish that task. We help the child to grow the neuronal structure of their brain, but what about the older adults in our society? The laws of neurogenesis and neuroplasticity are with us at all ages.

As long as you are alive the law of neuroplasticity will operate to maximize signaling between cells and conserve resources (blood) where it can. If blood is going to areas in the brain that aren't functioning the law of neuroplasticity will redirect it to an area that is functioning.

Neuroplasticity will kill off newly generated cells that are not used so that they don't consume blood and interfere with messaging. It will also kill off old cells that were once used, but are longer being used. These cells no longer have a value, and will be "pruned-off". Memory will begin to get worse. Eventually learning, reasoning, problem solving will be noticeably affected. As this is happening connections in the brain will be changing pushing us into a downward spiral. This process isn't immediate like "pruning" a bush or a tree. The brain is very careful about the cells that need to be "pruned". It takes its time. Time means aging which might help explain why "age" is blamed for cognitive decline.

The Need for Information

Your brain needs to know as much about its environment as is possible. Because of that need my brain, your brain, is responsive to the receipt of new information. My brain learned how not to speak because of the information it was receiving. Apparently, that information was strong enough to overcome my innate ability to speak. It also responded to the new information that allowed me to learn how to speak. My brain was constantly soaking up information based on what I was and wasn't doing. Based on the new information it was receiving it determined what was and wasn't needed and adjusted my behavior accordingly. Apparently, my brain had concluded that that was the way to survive. I knew that the brain was constantly processing information, but this put a twist on it. It allowed me to conclude that my brain had to be continually processing new information if I wanted to retain my cognitive abilities. The reason turned out to be relatively simple.

Eons ago, when the brain was just a fledgling trying to survive it had to be sure to avoid predators. It needed water and nutrition to survive. But to survive it needed to know where those things were that would allow it to avoid predators. It began to notice things it hadn't noticed before, and it started to understand what those things meant to its survival. That's where neurogenesis came in. Neurogenesis provided the cells needed to process and store the information. Neuroplasticity organized and rearranged things to provide the room in the brain needed to store the new cells and cellular networks. It also established new pathways and connections needed for communication.

The brain was receiving information about its environment and it was learning how to stay safe. As it learned it began to recognize what things in its environment threatened its survival, and what things helped to ensure its safety.

Up to this point the Primary Brain had the Emotional Sub-brain to help it out, but the Emotional Sub-brain was somewhat simplistic. It only responded in terms of safety, fight or flight.

As the environment in which the Primary Brain existed became increasingly complex the brain's need for new information grew, and the more complex the environment in which it existed the more new information it required. This increase in complexity and difficulty led to the development of the Logical, Executive Sub-brain with its box of cognitive tools. Those tools included perception, awareness of self, memory, learning, reasoning, and problem solving. More, such as the ability to engage in complex communications, evolved as time and need went on.

I know that it's rather strange to be talking about survival in our day and age, but the need to survive is still with us. The circumstances are much more complex, but if you think about it we need the same things that our earliest ancestor's needed. We need to avoid predators, people that threaten our survival. We need water and nutrition, and we need shelter. With the help of our cognitive tools the new information we receive tells us were we can find those things. That makes our brains responsive to new information.

Our cognitive tools serve us well as children, teenagers, and young adults. That's the time in our lives when we are continually receiving, processing and storing new information. We are learning! That's the time in our lives when we're expected to learn, and you can't learn without processing new information.

Neurogenesis is providing us with the new cells that we need. Neuroplasticity is establishing new cellular networks based on function, reorganizing and rearranging old ones, establishing new connections and laying down new pathways for communication. It's also establishing new arterial networks so that the new cells receive the blood they need.

It's a time in our lives when cells and cellular networks are nurtured. They're either pristine or relatively undamaged, and can function at optimum levels, but, as we age that changes.

Our brain cells are constantly being attacked by oxidants and toxins. Cells become inflamed, and some deplete with time and, most probably, use. The foods we eat and drink affect the condition of our brain cells. If we don't make the effort as we age, the health of our brain cells decline and along with it their ability to function as effectively as they did previously. It's our cognitive abilities that will take the hit, particularly memory. Since memory is key to all cognitive abilities, our cognitive functioning begins a steady, noticeable decline.

When this begins to happen you don't say that "…My brain is hurting…My brain is not healthy…" Your brain doesn't hurt. Your brain doesn't feel pain or discomfort. Unless there are some very obvious symptoms, you don't think about the health of your brain. It's just up there on your shoulders and you accept it for what it is. If it loses a step or two you think that it's just age.

You might feel irritable, recall of words might be more difficult, your memory might get sluggish or even bad, and your mental sharpness and agility might suffer. Any or all of these things might occur over time, but you don't think about your brain as being healthy or unhealthy, hurting or not hurting. I know I didn't. You chalk it up to age, and you begin to stay away from those things that test it. You reduce or stop processing new information. You stop learning, and you convince yourself that what you're doing, or not doing, is appropriate for someone your age. When we get older we're no longer expected to learn.

I was always under the impression that my brain functioned as effectively as it could all the time, regardless of age. Sure, I knew that toxic fumes and trauma could have some really negative effects on my brain. I also knew that the viral encephalitis I had took its toll, but that was about the extent of it.

It wasn't until I began to study the brain and those things that influence its functioning that I realized that my brain wasn't healthy. My ability to speak, or rather not to speak, had nothing to do with it. I taught myself how not to speak. As far as my brain was concerned it was doing the right thing. It was my bad memory, my reasoning ability and the difficulty that I had learning new things that should have told me that my brain was in trouble.

Once again I was fortunate, but my only choices were to either succumb to whatever it was that had trashed my memory and ability to speak, or try and repair them.

My disability had a major impact on my life. That disability was the motivating factor that pushed me, but if it had happened at any other time I might not have been as fortunate. It was motivation and timing that allowed me to learn how my brain functioned, what it needed to function effectively, and how to keep it healthy. At the top of that list was the processing of new information; learning new things. I was studying the brain and processing a lot of new information. My brain and I were both very happy.

Today it's common for adult children to encourage their older, adult parents to engage in mental exercises so that they can keep their brain healthy and functioning. I'm sure that you've heard the phrase "…Use it or lose it". Actually it should be "Use it and improve it…If you don't use it you'll lose it". That's true for people at any age, and the earlier in life they understand that the better.

Because of the word "exercise" people usually think of mental exercise as being puzzles, games, and mind stumpers. That's a very limiting interpretation of mental exercise. Mental exercise is anything that requires your brain to interact with, process, and learn NEW things.

Puzzles, games and mind stumpers are a good momentary effort. They can enhance focus, stretch your powers of perception and reasoning, and possibly increase processing speed if engaged in repeatedly over time. They keep your brain engaged and flexible. But puzzles, games and mind stumpers aren't going to do the job by themselves. For the most part, they have no importance or priority. They don't have anything to do with life content. Good mental exercise should involve visual or auditory input, memory, logic or reasoning, focus, **and it should have meaning**.

Good mental exercise should include things like learning a new job, learning to speak another language, learning to sign, learning to play a musical instrument, learning to cook, learning to paint, learning to dance, learning to operate a computer, learning a new software program, learning how to write effectively, learning to play golf, learning how to sing, learning math, learning a new skill of any kind. "LEARNING ANYTHING!".

To keep your brain healthy, both physically and functionally, and your cognitive skills sharp, you have to continue to learn new things throughout your life, regardless of age. If your brain is not receiving new information it will begin shutting down those areas that are not being used. This is primarily true of the areas in your Logical, Executive Sub-brain where learning, memory, reasoning, and problem solving are its primary functions.

The neat thing about your brain, thanks to the laws of neurogenesis and neuroplasticity, is that even though your cognitive abilities have declined they can be re-established, possibly even expanded. It all depends on what you do or don't do. The processing of new information and learning is a great place to start, but to do that you have to keep your brain, with its cells, pathways, neurotransmitters and connections, healthy.

The Stress Response!

There is something else related to information that needs to be understood about the cognitive functioning of your brain. That's the "stress response". We refer to it as just "stress". In actuality it's a response to information that's been received, possibly added to information that's been received over time, and processed through the Emotional Sub-brain.

To understand the "stress response" it's important to remember that information to the brain is anything that it receives from any of its five sensors that needs to be processed. Those sensors are vision, smell, hearing, taste, touch and feel. Only new information needs to be processed.

The "stress response" Came about as the brain's internal survival tool. New information about its environment would alert it to danger. I would imagine that it worked something like this: The Emotional Sub-brain would scan the environment looking for water, food, and shelter without interference from predators. The "stress response" would have been initiated by anything that threatened survival, a lack of food, too little water, bad weather, a sharp sound, unexpected movement, the presence of predators, anything.

If something was evaluated as a threat or a potential threat by the Emotional Sub-brain the Primary Brain was alerted, and the stress response was activated. That's how it worked back then and that's how it works now, although now it seems that the Logical Executive Sub-brain gets in the act as well.

As a survival tool the "stress response" was intended to be positive, and it can be if the response is focused and limited in duration. But the "stress response" can get out of control, particularly in our world. When it does it can be nasty and damaging to brain function, particularly cognitive function. When the "stress response" was first put into use the brain didn't think of it as being nasty or even potentially nasty. It just worked out that way. So, what happened?

When the "stress response" is activated two hormones, cortisol and adrenaline (epinephrine), are released into the circulating blood. Threats usually required a lot of attention and effort, even if it just meant getting away. A lot more energy was needed, and since sugar is the brain's primary source of energy, more sugar was needed. That's where adrenaline comes in. Adrenaline is an excellent sugar substitute.

Although adrenaline might appear to be the episodic hero, it's cortisol that takes charge as the System Manager. It's cortisol that holds back all internal systems not directly needed to deal with the stressor, even redirecting blood flow so that potential energy in the form of sugar and adrenaline can be directed at defeating or avoiding the stressor.

When this all started cognitive function didn't exist, and the "stress response" functioned for short periods of time. Increasing blood flow to those areas that needed it and holding back, or slowing, blood flow to other areas wasn't a problem. That's the way it worked back then and that's the way it works now but now we have a complex society with sophisticated forms of communication and the Logical Executive Sub-brain with its cognitive tools. Information is not just a literal interpretation of events. The Logical Executive sub-brain has a memory, holds on to, relates, and analyzes information that might present a threat. It passes its conclusions on to the Emotional Sub-brain for appropriate action. That's why the "stress response" can be a problem.

The brain can produce enough adrenaline to deal with short term stress. In fact, everything tends to work better if there are continuous repetitions of short term events that produce the "stress response". If the stress continues, along with the threat, or the perceived threat, that it presents, the adrenaline depletes leaving cortisol out there all by itself. The stressor still exists, adrenaline has been depleted and cortisol still has a job to do. So, it remains in place and tries to do what it can to defeat the stressor.

Unfortunately, cortisol's efforts are not well focused. It holds back systems that might be useful. It continues to hold back blood flow, possibly to the brain, and it attacks whatever it can. Rather than being a help the "stress response" and cortisol cause more problems.

The cortisol attacks nerve tissue, and causes cell damage that can affect cell function. The cortisol is toxic. At this point cortisol is playing two roles. It's still keeping the non-involved portions of the system in slow gear and it's trying to be the good guy that combats the stressor. It even shrinks the hippocampus, where new cells are generated for memory and learning, to avoid distraction. That reduces the number of new cells that can be generated and has a negative impact on memory and learning. It most likely reduces reasoning and problem solving abilities as well. Long term stress interferes with cognitive function, but the way in which the "stress response" functions is unique to the individual.

Each of us, as we grow and develop, has learned that certain things that could possibly be threats are tolerable occurrences that don't really threaten survival. We develop an acceptable threat level. Our stress response is not activated until we exceed that level. Understanding which potential threat is real and which potential threat can be tolerated is learned based on understanding and experience.

When a baby cries to be fed they've been threatened. They are under stress. In our country the child will most likely learn that hunger is not threatening. A child, adolescent or adult that wants to fit in with their peers feels threatened and is under stress. That's part of growing up. Having an assignment done correctly and on time raises the possibility of failure and can produce stress, depending on how it's handled. When you're in a competition you want to win. The desire to win or the thought of losing can create stress. They used to say that Arnold Palmer, the golfer, was such a good competitor because he had ice water in his veins. It's reasonable to assume that his "stress response" kicked in focusing his system, both cognitive and physical, on what had to be accomplished.

Being attractive and desirable to a member of the opposite sex presents the possibility of rejection. That can be stressful particularly in people with low self-esteem. Being in a battle zone is stressful even if you're protected. Performing in the workplace can be stressful or it can be acceptable, but so is making enough money to care for your family. If your family's well-being and survival are dependent on your ability to provide you could be under a lot of stress. If you have a certain life style that you feel you must live up to you are under stress. A person living in a neighborhood full of violence is under stress. Our environment, our health, our financial situation, our children, our wives, our bosses, even our friends can cause us to be stressed. The threat of being successful at something may not be life threatening, but it certainly can affect our quality of life.

Our acceptable stress levels result from repetitive stress situations that are resolved. We've learned that when they occur we don't have to worry. Our "stress response" doesn't kick in. Unexpected threats push us over that acceptable line. If it lasts too long it becomes a problem. Our "stress response" is based on what we experience and what we expect of ourselves.

We all must perform in some way. Based on our upbringing and experiences we establish our own expectations for performance. Making sure that we perform as expected is stressful. It doesn't matter if you're talking about being a quarterback on football team or having sex. Stress is all about life and what we want to get out of it at any point in time, at any age.

Stress is about the expectation of being able to survive in a comfortable state, however it is the individual defines comfort. Stress can be useful, kick your performance or response up a notch, or it can be damaging. It's really up to the individual. Stress will have an effect on the health and functioning of your brain. For the most part, it can be a positive or negative affect depending on how you perceive your environment. How you establish your normal stress level will depend on your upbringing, your experiences, and your understanding of what goes on around you. Short term stress will normally work for you. It's the circumstances that produce long term stress that you have to watch out for.

We develop a tolerance for "acceptable levels of stress", but stress is always with us. The health and functioning of your brain will depend on how you perceive your environment which will, in turn, determine how your stress response functions.

Your brain is your control center. It will continuously respond to what you do or don't do. You will be limited to doing what it can and can't do and it will control what you will and won't do. Just don't let your stress response get the better of you.

Section Three -

Effect OF What you eat and Drink

Oxidation, the Damage Doer

I was reading, studying, learning, all kinds of new things about my brain. Information didn't come from one place. It came from all over. I would find a thread and just follow it. It's amazing what things affect the health and functioning of your brain. That's when I came face to face with oxidation.

Oxidation is a cell killer. Oxidative stress, the result of oxidation, is a brain killer. Oxidative stress is considered to be a major factor in decreasing nerve-cell function and memory loss. In fact, there's been a lot of work done that points to oxidative stress as a prime cause of cognitive decline in aging.

When metal becomes rusty it's being oxidized. The oxygen, in the form of rust, is eating through the metal. We live in an atmosphere loaded with oxygen. We need to survive so we've adapted to the oxygen. That's weird since oxygen is one of the most corrosive gases in the universe. We try to keep the oxygen that we breath free of toxins, and we either protect the metal we have so that it won't rust or we develop a metal, like stainless steel, that doesn't succumb to the corrosive attacks of the oxygen.

When it comes to material we take steps to prevent oxidation. Most of us are not that caring or innovative when it comes to the brain. I know I wasn't. When you first think about it, it doesn't seem possible that oxygen could affect your brain the same way that it affects metal. But it does!

Your brain is soft tissue so it works a little differently. The cells in the brain need oxygen to function. It's the oxygen that allows the glucose (fuel) to fire so that the cell enzyme can use it as energy. But the oxygen doesn't just go away after it's used.

When oxygen is converted from fuel to energy it loses an electrical charge, becomes unbalanced and nasty. It becomes an oxidant. The oxidant strikes out and begins attacking healthy, balanced tissue looking to regain its electrical charge.

Those attacks damage tissue and cell function, but it doesn't stop there. Before the attack the molecules in the damaged tissue had balanced electrical charges. When the oxidant attacked it removed the balancing electrical charges, but molecules need to exist in an electrically balanced state. The damaged molecule goes from friendly and happy, doing its job, to unhappy and nasty unable to function. It replaces the attacking oxidant. The damaged, electrically unbalanced molecule starts attacking healthy tissue, electrically balanced molecules, looking to regain its lost charge and stability.

Unless these attacks are stopped it just keeps happening. Tissue and cells are damaged and lose functioning ability. That could mean that you lose some cognitive function. When I began to understand how this happened I pictured one molecule going out at a time, attacking and damaging other cells. That's not how it works.

Your brain contains approximately 100 billion brain cells. The cells that are working are constantly converting fuel into energy and producing free radical oxygen molecules otherwise known as oxidants. That army of oxidants is constantly attacking your brain tissues. That suggests that hundreds, thousands, millions, possibly billions of oxidants, are constantly being released into the environment where your brain lives and works. Those oxidants are attacking, ravaging and leaving a cascading trail of damage behind. The results is oxidative stress and damaged, poorly functioning cells.

When I understood what was taking place in my brain I actually began to feel sorry for it. I had neglected it, and even though it was doing its best, it was hurting. What had happened to my memory, and some of my other cognitive skills, was really my brain calling for help.

My brain was up there on my shoulders since birth. I had taken it for granted. I had assumed that it would always be with me, that my brain was what it was, and it was going to continue to be that way. As long as I avoided more head trauma it would be fine. I was wrong.

The Law of Neuroplasticity saw to it that the internal structure of my brain was constantly changing based on what I did and didn't do, but the damage that my diet had allowed to occur added another dimension to that. My brain was constantly changing based on what I did or didn't do, but it was also changing based on what it could and couldn't do. If it couldn't do something I avoided doing it.

I had neglected my brain reducing, possibly limiting, its functioning ability. That had a major impact on my life. What I was doing was being governed by what my brain could and couldn't do. That was an astounding realization. Talking, learning, reasoning and problem solving were all great examples. At that point I knew that I had to stop the damage doing. I had to eliminate the oxidants before they could do any more damage and, if possible, I had to begin healing the oxidative stress that had been building up all these years.

My brain cells, your brain cells, all healthy brain cells have a built-in defense force. That defense force is "glutathione". Glutathione is a "super" anti-oxidant. It attracts and eliminates oxidants before they can do any damage.

Unfortunately, the way we eat and what we eat overwhelms the defense capabilities of glutathione. It's like a fully equipped army overwhelming a poorly defended village. When that happens the oxidants are allowed to roam and ravage at will.

This wasn't recognized as a problem until recently. We didn't live long enough for it to be a problem. Our society wasn't as complex.

We didn't eat as much, and what we ate was much healthier. We didn't have the technology to understand what was going on and it was accepted that as you aged you lost cognitive ability. Oxidative stress had to be playing a major role in causing my cognitive problems.

Look Around You!

You might ask yourself "...If my brain is so smart why didn't it know all these things?" Good question! As it turns out, the brain originally did pursue and respond to those things that it needed in the environment in which it existed. But that environment goes way back and lasted for a very, very, long time. It was an environment where sweets were rare and there wasn't any processed food.

During that time we were physically active avoiding or defending against predators as well as trying to secure food, water and shelter. We were trying to learn about our environment. Our environment gave us water to drink, fruits and vegetables to eat, free range, grass fed meat, shelter, and we got plenty of sleep.

At the instruction of the brain we went after those things that were available, and those were the things that allowed the brain to feel safe. Those were the things that the brain learned and knew. If it could obtain what was available it would be safe. So it learned to go after what was available. It even rewarded itself for obtaining the things it needed to stay safe. Your brain still goes after what's available. Your brain still rewards itself when it gets something good, but the brain only knows what it knows.

The brain existed for a long, long time in that earlier environment, and that's the environment that it still knows, but the brain can learn. Unfortunately, because of the environment in which we live it's learning the wrong things.

In the last 100 years or so the environment has changed along with the availability of food, water and shelter. What the brain knows comes from vision, hearing, smell, taste, touch and feel. Have you looked around you lately?

Our environment consists of supermarkets with lots of processed foods, farm raised, grain fed, pen fattened beef, sugary drinks, fast food outlets with foods rich in saturated fat, fried foods, and more sugary drinks. There are television ads constantly blasting at us to consume more sugary drinks, eat more food with more saturated fat and cholesterol. They make it look good, sound good, and if you're in the vicinity, smell good.

My brain, your brain, is receiving the wrong information. It's being fooled into believing that the foods that are easily available in the surrounding environment are the foods that will help it to survive. In fact, a lot of the foods that are easily available and constantly promoted are damaging to the brain and its survival. I was eating them. I was damaging my brain and hurting its functioning ability.

The Importance of Metabolism

I had just started to understand the impact that food had on the functioning of my brain, both positive and negative. Then one evening I was at the Carnegie Institute of Washington attending a lecture. I had attended lectures there before but this was the first time I noticed this particular plaque on the wall. It read "Metabolism or Reproduction which came first?"

The answer had to be metabolism. Even at the very beginning the brain had to be the control center. If it was attempting to avoid predators by reproducing it needed energy and protein. They had to come from somewhere, and they had to be converted so the brain could use them. Whatever provided the energy and protein had to be metabolized so that it could be used. I was really pleased with myself for coming up with the answer and wanted to tell someone, but I was sure that they already knew.

Interestingly, I didn't give the metabolism interface much more than a nod at the beginning. After all, I was dealing with my brain not my stomach. I had always looked at digestion and metabolism as two separate things. My parents always told me that I had to chew my food really well so that it digested. They didn't tell me that I had to chew my food so that it metabolized well. But, at my age it was clear that digestion lead to metabolism.

Most people, including myself, looked at digestion and metabolism as two separate processes. I couldn't get my head around the two separate parts. To me the link between what I ate and what went into my blood had to be continuous but it didn't seem to be. To help me understand the process I relabeled things a bit, added a step, and put them all under the heading of Metabolism (capital "M"): a four part process. Part 1 was digestion, part 2 was sorting, part 3 was preparation, and part 4 was loading. The link was continuous, and I was able to relate the process to my brain.

I know that this all might seem a bit strange to you, but it's the way I made things work for me. The extraction and conversion process was metabolism but Metabolism, with a capital M, was also my Food Manager. He was responsible for managing what I ingested and seeing to it that it got to the right place at the right time. It was my job to get him the right materials.

I know that we consider eating to be something that's important to the functioning of our bodies, and it is. As I said in a previous chapter, I never connected eating and drinking with the health and cognitive survival of my brain. Now, I was learning that the brain's ability to survive and function is dependent on the foods we eat and drink. It was the sign at the Carnegie that made me take notice of the importance of converting that food and drink into elements that my brain needed to stay healthy and function effectively.

I needed to eat and drink foods that would keep my brain hydrated, provide it with a defense against oxidants, make sure that it had building blocks to repair, build and rebuild brain tissue, workers to get the job done, and useable energy. My brain needed all those things. That was the purpose behind eating and drinking. It was Metabolism's job to extract the needed ingredients from the food I ate and get them moving so that they could be delivered to the brain when it needed them. Everything else was secondary.

My food manager, Metabolism, was key to the health and cognitive survival of my brain, but there were limitations to what he could and couldn't do. The brain can't store fuel. It can't store anything. That meant that Metabolism had to get the needed ingredients to the brain when they were needed, but there were complications. The survival of the brain was Metabolism's primary responsibility, and the body portion of the Brain-body System needed the same ingredients, that meant that rationing was needed. Metabolism rationed and distributed the fuel received based on what the brain needed when.

The needs of the brain always came first. There always had to be enough for the brain. At best, the amount needed was a guess, but Metabolism had a memory it could rely on to get this done. The real issue was the food it had to work with, and that was beyond Metabolism's control. The brain had to provide it.

The brain went after what was easily available in its environment and the brain only knew what it knew. In my case that presented a problem for Metabolism. More rationing was needed. The primary ingredients to be rationed were water for hydration, fuel for energy and protein, the workers.

For my brain to function effectively, it needed to receive 20-25% of all the blood in my System. Actually, it needed to receive 20-25% of what my blood contained,, and that came primarily from the foods that I ate and drank. I didn't realize it until then, but the foods that I was eating and drinking were presenting a problem for my newly appointed Food Manager.

As long as I ate and drank the right foods and delivered them the right way, Metabolism's job was easy. But I wasn't eating or drinking the right foods, and that includes water. I wasn't at the extreme end of a bad diet, but it doesn't take much to walk near the edge. I wasn't helping my brain with what I was eating, and I certainly wasn't making my Food Manager's job any easier. I was trying to stop a slide in my cognitive abilities, but when it came to the foods that I was eating and drinking I wasn't helping. For me to regain my cognitive abilities I had to get my brain healthy again and that required the right foods.

When my cognitive problems started, I wasn't providing my Food Manager with enough water to keep my brain properly hydrated. I wasn't dehydrated but I'm sure that for those cells in my brain to work they had to suck every last bit of water out of their environment. I wasn't eating enough fruits and vegetables to build up my brain's defense force against oxidants, or Omega-3 unsaturated fat to be used as materials to repair and build tissue. I did okay in the Worker department with protein, and I was heavy on energy producing carbohydrates, but for the most part I was providing the wrong ones. It's hard to learn something and then ignore it, particularly if you're working on a related problem. Your brain knows what it knows, and now it knew what it needed.

You are constantly placing demands on your system internally and externally, but it's the trillions of living, functioning cells, throughout the Brain-body System, each with a task, that are actually doing the work. They need all of the same things that the brain needs.

The cells and cell networks in your Brain-body System need to be kept hydrated and fed. They need a defense force to protect them against oxidants, building material to repair and rebuild cells, workers to put things together, energy to make it all happen, and waste to be removed. Metabolism is constantly monitoring all of this activity, determining what each cell needs to accomplish its given task, and relating that to what it has to work with.

In primitive times, eons ago, food and the fuel derived from it were scarce. Even though food in this country is in abundance your brain looks back and recognizes that food can become scarce. When something is scarce you don't want to waste it. You want to use it efficiently. Your brain is the same way. It doesn't want to waste fuel so it has Metabolism balance all of the food that it's receiving with the functioning requirements of the entire Brain-body System. That means that what goes into your blood must be balanced with need.

To assess need with fuel availability Metabolism has to be constantly monitoring the activities of the Brain-body System for fuel requirements. It delivers that fuel in your circulating blood. But it just can't load everything into your blood for delivery. Metabolism has to be constantly balancing the availability of food and water, and the fuel content of that food, with the need for fuel.

I began to realize that I was driving my Food Manager up a wall with what I was eating and drinking. I had to give my food manager and my brain a good chance of being successful. That would only happen if I changed my diet.

Your brain is working all the time, 24 hours a day. It needs a constant stream of fuel deliveries. The rest of the Brain-body System takes off when you're sleeping but your brain keeps on working.

Other than when you're sleeping the trillions of living, functioning cells, each with a task, is placing demands on Metabolism's fuel supply. The cells in your Brain-body System need to be kept hydrated and fed. They need a defense force to protect them against oxidants, building material to repair and rebuild cells, workers to put things together, energy to make it all happen, and the waste to be removed. Metabolism is constantly monitoring all of this activity and determining what each cell needs to accomplish its given task.

For Metabolism to make the right decisions it relies on memory. It has to go back to what was needed in the past and what was provided to fulfill those needs. Metabolism has to determine, if things go as they have, whether the available fuel will be scarce or plentiful. If fuel is scarce Metabolism will short some of the less needy cells while storing some of the fuel it receives for future use.

If fuel is abundant, and there is more than is needed, Metabolism has no needy customers to send it to. That excess will go into storage as fatty acid for future use, but converting it back into fuel will be inefficient and take time. The future need for energy will not be met quickly if there is reliance on storage fat.

It gets even more complicated! Metabolism has to have some way of determining what's needed and what's available, particularly when it comes to the brain. It does this by monitoring and regulating temperature. Yes, temperature!

Each of the foods that you provide have potential heat and energy in the form of calories. When those calories are burned that potential heat becomes actual heat. That heat produces the energy needed by the cell to perform a function. Carbohydrates and fats have an energy potential of 9 calories per gram; protein has an energy potential of 4 calories per gram.

Temperature then becomes a convenient measure of how much energy is needed and how much fuel should be sent to a functioning location in the Brain-body System, including the brain. It also tells Metabolism how much of what's available needs to be stored as fat. The available ingredients that are not sent to a functioning location in the Brain-body System are converted to fat, and sent to storage for future use. Where it goes depends on available space.

Remember, historical data informed Metabolism that the brain needed 20 – 25% of the converted (metabolized) food. But the brain can't store fuel. The brain has to use fuel, for whatever purpose, pretty much, as it's received. It then has to balance that fuel with function or need. A big part of Metabolism's job is to see that the brain and other parts of the Brain-body System get only the fuel that they need. Taken all together, that's a lot of work. But Metabolism has a weakness.

Foods don't enter the blood all at the same time or at the same rate. The different types of foods have different conversion times. Entry into the blood is a gradual process. At least, it's supposed to be. That doesn't always happen with carbs, since Metabolism can't tell the difference between good carbs and bad carbs. Metabolism can't tell the difference between carbs that convert and enter the blood gradually and carbs that convert and enter the blood quickly. To Metabolism a carb is a carb, and a carb contains 9 calories per gram of potential energy. All carbs, whether simple or complex, are converted into glucose and sent out for distribution either as energy or as storage fat.

The gradual distribution of fuel is extremely important to the brain, the control center of the Brain-body System. Since the brain can't store fuel, it needs to receive fuel gradually as needed. Carbs convert to glucose. Brain cells convert that glucose to energy. That would work well if all carb's entered the System gradually, but that's not what happens.

Typically, it's the fiber in a carbohydrate (carb) that slows its conversion to glucose allowing it to enter the blood and delivered to the brain gradually. Simple carbs do not have much, if any fiber. They don't contain anything that will slow the conversion process. Although all carbs are glucose (metabolized sugar), simple carbs enter the blood about 15 times faster than complex carbs. Too much sugar (simple carbs) enters the blood at one time. That causes sugars (glucose) to be delivered in excessive quantities and burned much more quickly than needed. Sugar delivery in large amounts is great when you're running a race, lifting weights, or something similar. When you're doing those things you need lots of energy. If not, all that sugar creates a problem for Metabolism and the brain.

Simple carbs, simple sugars, fool Metabolism into believing that there's more fuel available for use than there actually is. More quick carbs are allowed to enter at one time. Healthier foods are blocked and more fuel goes into producing toxic waste and storage fat. But that's not all that happens. Simple carbs create an energy void.

Metabolism's primary responsibility is the brain's survival. Because the glucose from simple carbs enters the blood quickly and in excessive quantities too much is delivered too quickly to the brain to be useable. Metabolism thinks that the brain has more useable energy than it does so it slows down its deliveries. In the meantime a slew of unnecessary oxidants are produced overwhelming the brain's internal defenses, creating tissue inflammation, and damaging cell function. When this happens the brain can become sluggish, slowing function.

When I started I thought that the primary objective of Metabolism was to move food into my blood. The more I learned the more that changed. Metabolism's primary objective is to make sure that the brain has fuel in times of need and scarcity. It manages the food that it receives accordingly.

If fuel is readily available, and easily obtainable in relation to perceived need, then Metabolism will put more fuel into storage for future use. That fuel goes in storage as a fatty acid somewhere in the body. The opposite is true as well. If fuel is not readily available the needs of the brain will take priority and fuel will be conserved so that it's available when needed by the brain. That can make you feel sluggish.

That suggests that if there is a small, steady, flow of the right foods going to Metabolism it can balance the need for fuel with the fuel that it's receiving more easily. Energy can be kept at optimum levels. Toxic waste can be eliminated more easily. There will be less damage as a result of oxidation. Your brain will be healthier, and your cognitive abilities will function much better.

I thought that I knew the importance of eating and drinking the right foods. But it was understanding the role of Metabolism that wrapped everything into a neat package. Once I was able to put everything together I could make the connection between the foods I was eating and drinking and my brain, particularly my ability to function cognitively. Understanding the role and importance of Metabolism provided me with the insight that I needed to truly understand what my diet and lack of proper hydration had been doing to the health of my brain.

If I was going to get my brain back into a healthy state I needed to eat foods in a way that would provide building materials, workers and energy in a balance that Metabolism could work with easily. I needed to eat the right foods in small quantities throughout the day.

Healing my Forgiving Brain

It wasn't all bad. In fact, the outlook was quite promising. I was learning that although my brain was incredibly complex it was also very forgiving. But I had to stop the damage that I was doing to my brain as a result of my diet. I had to provide it with those foods that would allow it to heal. The most damage was being caused by simple carbohydrates or simple sugars. They were the primary cause of the oxidation that was taking place, but the way I was eating was causing a lot of the damage as well.

I was eating pretty much like everyone else. I ate breakfast, lunch and dinner, but I didn't like skimpy meals. They weren't excessive except on holidays. I learned as a child that if you wanted to stay healthy you have to eat. Do you remember the stories about the starving children in India, Africa, China or whatever location your folks used to get you to finish what was on your plate. I certainly did.

Like most other folks I was eating in fits and starts. I'd eat a decent meal. Then I wouldn't eat anything until the next big meal except, that is, when I snacked. I never really thought much about my eating or my snacking because I wasn't fat. I was overweight but I wasn't fat. I liked a good cheeseburger and fries for lunch, and I was addicted to Chicago hot dogs. They come with fries as well, and you can't eat hamburgers or hot dogs without some type of soda which, more than likely, was a sugary drink. Even with all that, I had convinced myself that my diet was on the healthy end of the scale.

My snacking occurred between meals and usually involved some type of candy or pastry, both of which are simple carbs. I might have been about 13 lbs. overweight, but that wasn't so bad as long as I didn't let it get any worse. Something I knew I could do. In my mind what I was eating was relatively healthy. I had no idea that I was damaging my brain and limiting its ability to function. I had to do something about it.

It wasn't that I just had to reduce the amount of food that I was eating. I had to start eating the right foods in the right way. The perplexing part is that I thought I was doing just that. I knew that this was going to require a big change in what I was eating and the way in which I was eating it. I hadn't even focused on hydration yet, although I have to say that it was always in the background.

I was focused on that little guy I had taken down off my shoulders *"my damaged, hurting brain"*. What did I need to do to fix him up? To start with, I was overwhelming the anti-oxidant capability of my brain with the amount and type of food that I was eating. I had to cut out or, at least, cut way back on simple carbs (simple sugars). They metabolized too quickly overwhelming my brain's internal defenses. I had to start eating so that what I was eating was of maximum benefit to my brain, and I had to strengthen my brain's ability to fight off oxidants. My diet had to contain more foods rich in anti-oxidants. They would act as my brain's defense force. That's where I planned to start. It wasn't going to be easy.

I loved fruit juice and sugar coated cereals. What they refer to as *"frosted"*. Most of those cereals, particularly the ones that I liked, not only had a sugar coat but were produced with refined wheat flour, both simple carbs (simple sugars). As if that wasn't enough, I would usually start off with some type of fruit juice and finish with coffee and a sweet pastry. I had no idea that I was starting my day on a sugar high. Sugar not only pumps you up but it brings you down as well. That prompts you to look for more sugar. By 10:00 I was ready for a snack, or as they like to call it, "a coffee break". That usually involved more coffee and some type of sweet pastry, normally a doughnut, possibly two. That was the sugar fix that would probably take me through until lunch.

Your Relationship with Food

Everyone has a relationship with the foods that they eat and drink. I know I did, and that relationship began when I was a child. I was raised in Chicago, and I had been eating Chicago Hot Dogs with salty fries, and drinking root beer since I was old enough to ask for it. That's who I was. Changing that relationship was not going to be easy.

Your relationship to food and eating has four components, and I never thought about any of them. Those components are emotional, intellectual, environmental and physical.

Your emotions as they relate to eating are strong. It's not only about what you ate as a child and "feeling good". Eating is about you and who you've been. If you change that you'll feel like you're changing who you are. That's the tough part to overcome. You have a built-in, emotional defense against changing what you eat.

You've been eating things that you like and avoiding things that you don't like for a lot of years. You've built up a menu of foods, good and bad, that you search out. Changing that is not easy. You like those foods, but a number of the foods you like are simple carbs. They're simple sugars. Your brain is addicted to that sugar and you like foods containing sugar.

I'll say it again, making that change is tough. I wasn't alone on an island doing whatever I wanted. I had to change. But that change would only come about if I could assimilate with my environment. After all these years, that was going to be tough.

My Logical Executive Sub-brain had learned why it was hurting and understood what had to be done. That was the intellectual phase, but before I could make any changes my Emotional Sub-brain had to be convinced that it wouldn't threaten my survival. That sounds silly, but I needed to accept the change emotionally. I had to understand and accept that even if I did make a big change to my eating I was still going to be me. I was just going to be a better, sharper, healthier me that would probably live longer.

It's a good guess that you're eating habits are fairly similar to those of your family and friends. Changing your eating habits will make you different. It's also reasonable to assume that you're exposed to the same type of stores, fast food outlets and advertising that they are. If you put your family and friends together with that surrounding infrastructure you have the environmental part of eating. If I hadn't had big time support and encouragement from my wife, who obviously makes up a big part of my environment, it's unlikely that I would have been able to make the needed changes to my diet.

Finally, there's the physical part. Everything about changing your eating habits is tough, but the physical part is not only tough it's sneaky. You can always justify eating the bad foods. That justification could be anything from *"I feel bad". I need some good foods to comfort me,"* to *"It won't hurt just this one time. What I eat is normally healthy,"* to the cravings produced by simple sugars.

Sugar is sugar, and the brain considers sugar to be a survival food. It makes no difference if you're eating an excess of complex carbs or a candy bar. Sugar is sugar, and unless you understand that intellectually and emotionally you will continue to consume sugar and lots of it. At first just a little, but it will escalate. You need to control your intake of carbs, particularly simple carbs or simple sugars.

Simple sugars are the worst. They hit the brain the fastest in the greatest quantities. They produce the biggest high and the lowest low. They also produce the worst oxidation.

Your brain wants the sugar high to continue. It craves sugar and it will continue to want more sugar. Sugar is an opiate to the brain, but like all opiates there's a downside. Simple sugars produce the highest concentration of oxidants, the worst oxidation and oxidative damage. That's physical. Getting rid of simple sugars is not easy, but if you understand why you need to get rid of them and have some will-power you can do it.

I still fight that battle. Most of the time I win, but there are still times when I lose. I don't dwell on it. I just know that it's tremendously important to the health and functioning of my brain to minimize the simple sugars I ingest and the amount of food that I eat at one time.

The Need to be Hydrated

I had a lot to do, and I needed a place to start. Hydration seemed to be the easiest thing to do and the best place to start. It didn't seem that getting and staying hydrated would be all that difficult. It was something I could handle so I focused my efforts on hydration. .Looking back, if I had started by trying to eliminate simple sugars there's a good chance it wouldn't have worked out.

Don't let me mislead you. Staying properly hydrated is incredibly important to the functioning of your brain. Your brain tissues and cells live in water. It's water that contains the foods that your brain feeds on. It's water that allows the cell enzymes to function. It's water that keeps the tissue and cells flexible and functioning. It's water that removes the waste and toxins, and its water that protects the brain from banging into that hard, bony, spiked thing that we refer to as a skull. No question, water is not only important it's critical.

When you think of staying properly hydrated it's no stretch to realize that means water. The obvious thing to do is to drink more water. At first, I tried drinking 8 ounces of water about every hour. That didn't work too well. I would get distracted, involved, wasn't anywhere I could get water or simply forgot, so I changed tactics.

I filled a 2 liter bottle with water. Instead of taking my water from the tap I took it from the refrigerated bottle. I seldom came close to emptying the bottle by dinner time. That meant that I had to drink whatever water was left in the bottle that evening. Since you're using water throughout the day and depleting your supply, that doesn't help much, and it's not the thing to do for a good night's sleep. You want to stop drinking about 3 hours before you go to bed.

Finally, I just made water my drink of choice. I stopped drinking other liquids until drinking water was just part of who I was. That seemed to work. I had established a relationship with water, and it didn't take more than a few weeks to kick my old drinking habits.

My water gauge told me when I was properly hydrated and when I needed more water. My water tank was my blood. The gauge was my urine and the indicator was the color of my urine. It's not a pleasant subject, but it's important. The color of urine tells you a lot about your level of hydration.

The water circulating in your system is bringing nutrients and salts to your brain. That's how it works on the way in. After the water has dropped off its cargo it leaves, but it doesn't leave empty-handed. The used water leaves with the waste that your brain cells have produced. That waste includes oxidants and toxins. Those oxidants and toxins are in a water solution. That water solution is treated internally with an acid.

You now have a solution of water, toxins, waste and acid that your blood is carrying on its way out. That solution is urine. The indicator that you have to pay attention to is the color of that urine. The darker the color of that urine the greater the percentage of waste, toxin and acid to water, and the lower your hydration gauge. To get that gauge up you want the solution to be as clear or as close to clear as possible. That means you want to add more water to the solution.

At this point, I was simply adding more water by drinking it, but there was still something that wasn't right. The color of my urine was changing throughout the day and evening. The up-down-up-down movement of my hydration indicator was driving me nuts. It just shouldn't be that way.

Then I realized, as I should have all along, that my level of hydration wasn't just the result of how much water I was drinking. It was much more complicated than that. My hydration gauge was reflecting what I was drinking, as well as what I was eating and doing, primarily how mentally and physically active I was and the amount of stress I was under.

Most water that you get from the foods you eat comes from fruits and vegetables. You get some from complex carbs and precious little, if any, from simple carbs. It all works together. My level of hydration was reflecting the functioning effectiveness of my system with my brain at the controls.

Understanding that drinking, eating and what I was doing didn't just help me hydrate all those brain cells so they could function more effectively. My venture into hydration got me focused on what I was eating and stopping the damage-doing. There are times when my indicator slips down because I'm not drinking enough, eating the right things or I'm under a lot of stress. When that happens I need to make the color correction by drinking more water, eating some fruit or salad, or removing myself from the stress situation I'm in. Hydration levels were helping me with what I was doing.

I stopped being concerned about the changing color of my urine throughout the day and paid more attention to what I was doing, when I was drinking water and what I was eating.

Overall my indicator was going up. My urine was getting lighter. There were even times when it was almost clear. I started looking for a color consistency. My objective was to get my urine to have less color each day (raise the indicator) until I had gotten it to the point where it was clear or almost clear.

With my understanding of Metabolism and hydration I started eating small amounts of the right foods throughout the day. I also kept a small bowl of grape tomatoes, carrots and sugar snap peas on my desk and I would periodically eat a piece of fruit. Eating that way allows your system to use what you eat with minimum waste and maximum benefit and that affects your level of hydration.

My hydration indicator stayed at higher levels, I felt better, my regular meals were smaller, and my weight started heading downwards. Now my weight hovers around what I weighed when I was a senior in college.

I still drank more water than I did before, but my drinking wasn't regimented, and I certainly didn't have to make sure that I drank a glass of water every hour. Water was my drink of choice and with the change in my eating I was getting all the water I needed.

Now, I'm relaxed about what I drink. There's always water, but I'll periodically have a cup of decaf coffee or decaf tea when I'm out. I drink water, vegetable juice and almond milk (unsweetened). When I'm at home I've replaced coffee with hot chocolate. I use dark, baking chocolate and add one teaspoon of sugar. It's great.

More Damage Doers, Trans Fats
and Added Sugar

I was feeling great. I was doing a lot. My diet was beginning to change. Whether it was the fact that I knew I was doing something to help or something was actually happening I can't say, but I was feeling good about it all, and I was feeling a lot sharper. I wanted to keep moving forward. I knew that I had to keep working at stopping the damage-doing. I needed to stop the oxidation that was taking place in my brain. I needed to eliminate, or at least minimize, my intake of simple sugars, the primary culprit.

While my brain and I were wrestling with simple sugars and hydration my wife became very concerned about trans-fats. Because trans-fats are not a natural fat your body has trouble clearing them. They remain and build-up as plaque on your blood vessels. Even ingesting small amounts is not good for you.

If you look on the serving label it will always say *"trans-fat 0"*. If you look on the ingredient label you never see trans-fats listed. Even so, the product you're looking at may contain trans-fat. Trans-fats are listed on the ingredients label as partially hydrogenated or hydrogenated oil, and it can be any type of oil. Trans-fats don't have to be listed on the serving portion of the label until they exceed 0.5 grams per serving. As a result, my wife and I made it a habit to read the ingredient labels on processed foods. We never purchase anything containing partially hydrogenated or hydrogenated oil.

One day my wife was reading the ingredient label on a package of hot chocolate we had purchased and she posed a question. "How do you know how much sugar the actual food contains and how much sugar has been added?" The answer is simple, but the question was pure genius. *"If there is no added sugar then the sugar is coming from the food."* It seems obvious that if no sugar is added it must be coming from the food, but it's something we never really thought about. Yet it's incredibly important if you're trying to stop the damage-doing and build a healthy brain.

By asking the question she focused attention on *"added sugars"* in foods. Once that question was asked we couldn't put it back in the bottle. The brain knows what the brain knows. Now it knew that processed foods containing added sugars were most likely not brain healthy. It may not seem like much, but there are foods that you would never suspect as having added sugar. Whole wheat, or whole grain, bread is a good example.

There was a whole-grain, sandwich bread that we purchased at a local, chain supermarket. With the exception of that whole grain sandwich bread, we normally just purchased non-food items there. The market where we normally purchased our food also sold a whole-grain bread. We didn't like their bread nearly as much so we didn't buy it.

When we read the ingredient labels on both breads we understood why. There was added sugar in the whole grain bread we liked. It was the sugar in the loaf of bread that caused us to say "we liked it better".

That question my wife had asked focused our attention on "added sugars" in packaged foods, and it was making a difference. Even the most unsuspecting packaged foods frequently contain added sugar to enhance the taste. The added sugars are usually identified on the ingredient label as some type of syrup, juice, sucrose, fructose, lactose, honey, maltose, molasses, or distilled sugar water.

Added sugar is simply there for taste, a taste that most of us have learned to "want" as a child. By eliminating, or minimizing, the use of packaged foods with added sugar, I would be cutting back on my sugar consumption even more. That meant less oxidation, less damage-doing. It's not as hard to do as you might think. After a short time you'll wonder why you ever ate sweetened, apple sauce or whatever processed foods with added sugar that you've been purchasing. If you want to add sugar to something to enhance the taste do it yourself. That way you know exactly how much sugar was added and you can add the minimum amount needed.

More about Simple Sugars

By this time I was on a hydration program. I had started eating small amounts of food every two to three hours. My intake of anti-oxidants had gone way up, building my brain's defense forces against oxidants. Anti-oxidants typically come from fruits and vegetables so I was getting more vitamins and minerals as well, a win-win situation all the way around. But I still had some major work to do.

Simple carbs aren't just refined sugars, candy and pastry. Simple carbs are any food product made from white flour, refined white flour, even enriched white flour. That meant no more white bread or bagels made the old fashioned way. I was a closet eater of a "Frosted" cereal. No more. Not only did it have a "sugar" coating it was made with white flour.

I grew up on white bread sandwiches as did a lot of other kids. That was at a time when people didn't know that products made with white flours weren't as healthy as products made with whole-grain flours. In fact they had no nutritional benefit. Even enriched flours fell far short of what whole-grain flours provide.

White flour is refined wheat flour that has had the bran and germ removed. That's why it's white. But the bran and germ are the healthy part of the wheat. Refined, even enriched, refined wheat, is a simple carb. It's nothing but sugar. A good portion of the energy it provides can't be used. When you eat foods made with white flour you will put excess sugar in your blood causing a sugar spike, overwhelming the brain's defenses against oxidants, and damaging cells. Keep that up long enough and it can affect cognitive function.

To stop more of the damage doing I switched to bread products made from whole grain. You would be surprised at the number of products made from refined flour that you eat in a day; sandwich bread, bagels, crackers, pasta, waffles, pancakes, pizza, and cereals to name a few.

Our breakfast is either an oat cereal with fruit and berries or an egg and wheat toast. We will periodically add some type of melon. There are all kinds of oat cereals; flakes, rounds, oatmeal. Eating them with some fruit or berries replaced the sugar I was ingesting, was brain healthy, and helped to prevent "cravings".

There was an issue about fiber. Fiber doesn't get digested and has no nutrient value. It's eliminated, but it's the fiber in the food product that allows all the good stuff to be metabolized and enter the blood gradually. Some whole grain sandwich breads are very rich in fiber. Their taste is unusual to say the least, but if that's what you like, it's fine. We had a bit of a problem with it so we drew the line at whole-grain breads heavy in fiber. That still left us with plenty of good, whole grain sandwich breads to choose from.

While all of this was going on I realized that stores were promoting "wheat" breads and "multi-grain" breads. I assumed that they were attempting to convince people that they were healthy. All bread is made from "wheat". Unless it's whole-grain wheat you're not getting any of the nutrients. The same is true of multi-grains. If those grains are not whole-grain you can have one of every type of grain, but it still won't be healthy. If it's whole wheat it will tell you on the ingredient label.

It seemed to me that with everything else that I was doing, minimizing simple sugars had pretty well stopped the damage doing. It probably didn't stop it all together, but it brought it down to an absolute, manageable, minimum. My list of simple carbs and damage doers included refined sugars, candy, pastry and products made from white flour and processed foods with added sugar.

I was doing way less damage to my brain. My brain was still producing oxidants but the oxidants were being produced in smaller amounts and spread out in time. That allowed my internal anti-oxidant glutathione, along with the anti-oxidants I was ingesting, to take care of those pesky oxidants before they could do much damage. And for the most part, I was staying properly hydrated, but I wasn't finished.

Brain Healthy Foods we Need

Foods are generally classified as 1) protein, 2) carbohydrate, and 3) fat. All foods fall into 1 or more of those 3 categories. Unfortunately, that doesn't tell you very much about the foods you should be eating and drinking to keep your brain healthy. It certainly didn't tell me very much so I decided to make it easier for myself by reclassifying foods.

My reclassification focused on what I needed to eat and drink and why. I included water as a food. The foods that I needed to eat and drink to keep my brain healthy fell into five categories. Those five categories are:

1) Water to keep my brain hydrated;

2) Anti-oxidants to support my brain's defense force.

3) Unsaturated fatty acids, particularly Omega-3 fatty acids, materials needed to heal, repair and build tissue.

4) Protein, my brain's worker-bees. They got things done.

5) Complex carbohydrates for the energy to make things happen.

ABOUT FAT

Now, I was ready! I had built a defense force and stopped the damage-doing. I felt good knowing that my brain was getting healthier. I also knew that the cells that had been damaged had to be repaired. New cells needed building materials, and since brain cells deplete with time and use they will need some type of uplift periodically. Even healthy cells need to be repaired and rebuilt from time to time. That's where fats or fatty acids come in. They're the building blocks, but fat isn't just fat.

There are "essential" and "non-essential" fatty acids. There are saturated fats and unsaturated fats, and then of course, there's cholesterol. Fats that are ingested and metabolized go into your blood as fatty acids. My initial assumption was that "essential" fatty acids were those that I needed and "non-essential" fatty acids were those that I didn't need. I was wrong.

That takes us back to Section Two "The Functioning Brain" and the part where I introduced "The Rules That Guide the Functioning of the Brain". Rule 5 reads

"The internal and external elements that the brain uses grow, or change, as the survival requirements of the brain grow, or change."

That rule introduces the Brain-body System with the brain as the control center. In essence, the brain develops what it needs to survive.

My brain, your brain, needs fatty acids for the repair and building of cells. The brain evolved an internal system in the body capable of making some of the fatty acids it needed. As I learned, the fatty acids that the Brain-body System produced on its own were classified as "non-essential". That simply meant that I didn't need to eat foods that contained the fatty acids that my system produced. My Brain-body System took care of most of it.

The "non-essential" fatty acids that my system produced internally were saturated fatty acids and cholesterol which is a steroidal fat. My brain needed both of these fatty acids and had evolved an internal system to produce them. Your internal system satisfies that need by producing most of what it needs from the foods that you eat.

Excess amounts of saturated fat are warehoused as storage fat somewhere on your body. Excess amounts of cholesterol get deposited on the inside of your blood vessels which is not good. It can slow or block blood flow. The next thing I learned really surprised me.

Saturated fat doesn't have any cholesterol, but your brain ties saturated fatty acids and cholesterol together in some way. When you ingest foods that contain saturated fat it will cause your system to produce cholesterol whether you need it or not. It's likely that the unneeded cholesterol produced will get deposited on your blood vessels as plaque. That will reduce or block blood flow.

Blood is the brain's primary resource. People get all upset about the possibility of blood clots and with good reason. Blood clots not only reduce cognitive function they can be fatal. You don't want a reduction in blood supply caused by partial blockages either. A reduction in blood supply can affect brain function, produce dizziness, disorientation and a loss of cognitive ability. My brain was in enough trouble. It didn't need to have its supply of blood shorted. I couldn't let that happen.

Unless you're a vegetarian it's almost impossible to completely avoid eating foods that contain, at least, some saturated fat. What you can do, though, is minimize the amount of saturated fat and cholesterol that you ingest, and that's what I did. Minimizing the saturated fats and cholesterol that I ingested was a change, but not all that difficult to make.

You normally have choices with the foods you eat. They're there if you look for them. For example, sweet potato with lemon and pepper instead of a baked potato with butter and sour cream, 1% milk instead of whole milk, baby carrots and sugar snap peas instead of M&M's, fish or a salad instead of farm raised, grain fed beef, Manhattan clam chowder instead of New England clam chowder, whole grain pretzels instead of potato chips, cut-up oranges instead of cookies or pastry, a chicken or turkey sandwich on whole grain bread instead of a hamburger on refined wheat bread, whole grain toast instead of a doughnut, and so on.

I can't say it enough. I felt like a new person, and I felt really good about what I was doing. I had stopped the damage doing, but as I learned my brain needed "essential" fatty acids to help it heal and rebuild.

"Essential" fatty acids are those that my Brain-body System needed but couldn't produce on its own. I needed to eat the foods that provided them. Essential fatty acids are metabolized unsaturated fats.

Unsaturated fatty acids have all of the structural components that work well for tissue construction everywhere in the body except the brain. As it turns out the brain is fussy about what it receives and when it receives it.

Prior to birth the brain uses the saturated fatty acid that it produces to build tissue, but that changes at birth. The brain still needs fatty acid but now it needs unsaturated fatty acid which the Brain-body System can't produce on its own and the brain can't store it. The brain can't store anything.

To continue to build new cells, to repair and rebuild tissue the brain needs unsaturated fatty acid which is an essential fatty acid. The Brain-body System can't produce it. All unsaturated fatty acids have the capability of repairing and rebuilding tissue but the brain is unique. It can't use just any unsaturated fatty acid. The only unsaturated fatty acids that it can use are in the Omega class of fatty acids; Omega-3 (O-3) and Omega-6 (O-6).

The brain can't store anything so it has to use what it receives fairly quickly. Omega fatty acids metabolize quickly which was why the brain can make use of them. I was confused.

The fat that I ingested was metabolized as a fatty acid when it entered my blood. Then it got through to me. At this point, all I needed to understand about metabolism was that it was a "*conversion process.*"

Omega fats were metabolized into my blood as a fatty acid, but when they reached my brain they were metabolized a second time into different acids that my brain cells could receive. Cells in the brain have receptors for certain elements. Those are the only elements that those cells can receive and use. Brain cells will receive the component elements of Omega-3 and Omega-6 fatty acid. Unfortunately the cell receptors that receive Omega-3 and Omega-6 are the same ones, and that's not good.

The brain needs fatty acid to heal, repair and build tissue. We need both Omega fatty acids in the Brain-body System, but that presents a problem. They can both be used as building material but other than that they do different things. Omega-3 has an anti-inflammatory ability and heals and builds tissue. Omega-6 strengthens the immune response by producing inflammation and encouraging blood clotting.

That may not sound like much of a difference but it's actually the difference between a healthy brain and a hurting brain. The tissue inflammation response produced by Omega-6 fatty acid is intended to be protective, but it interferes with cell function. Not only that, our diets normally provide much more Omega-6 than Omega-3. That's because Omega-6 is much more prevalent in the foods we eat.

At first I didn't understand why this was a problem. Then I found out that too much Omega-6 in the diet will block the receptors needed by Omega-3 fatty acid. That meant that even if I stopped the damage-doing without Omega-3 fatty acid it was unlikely that I could heal and rebuild my brain tissue.

Without even realizing it I was well on my way to establishing a brain-healthy relationship between Omega-3 and Omega-6. I had already eliminated farm raised, grain fed, red meat from my diet as well as simple carbs and refined oils, and we seldom used processed foods anymore. Those are the primary sources of Omega-6. What I needed to do now was to increase my intake of those foods that were rich in Omega-3 polyunsaturated fatty acid and I wasn't far from doing it.

We had already made legumes, citrus fruit, melons and green leafy vegetables like broccoli, kale and spinach a regular part of our diet. The only thing that we needed to do was to increase the amount of cold water fish that we were eating and maybe add some flax seed to salads and cereal every now and then.

Before we made any changes to our diet my wife and I would eat salmon or tuna periodically, but not regularly. When we realized that we needed to increase our intake of Omega-3 fatty acid we made a conscious effort to have some type of cold water fish at least twice a week. With tuna and salmon on salads and sandwiches it was probably more often.

I had never eaten sword fish before. What a treat! And Cod fixed Portuguese style is excellent. It took me two months looking at a can of sardines in my refrigerator before I got up the nerve to try them. I should have gotten up the nerve to try them a lot earlier. I found that sardines on whole grain bread with honey mustard, onion, and tomato is just outstanding.

It was flax seed that caused a problem, but only because I didn't take the time to learn how to use them. First, flax seed has to be crushed to be beneficial. You can buy it that way, which I prefer, or you can crush them yourself. The next thing that you need to know about flax seed is that your system has to get used to it. Crushed flake seed on salads and cereals works really well if you start off slowly. A tablespoon of flax seed a day is really all you need, but start out by adding one-half a teaspoon and building gradually to a full tablespoon. You'll reap the rewards without the pain.

PROTEIN

I haven't mentioned protein, not directly anyway. Your brain needs protein. Your cells need protein to function and it's protein that facilitates the signaling between cells. I'm not sure where I stood on the protein scale. I was eating a fair amount of turkey breast and chicken breast, both excellent sources of protein. Cold water fish not only provides you with Omega-3 fatty acid it's a good source of protein, then there's eggs. Eggs have always been part of my diet, and they're listed in the top ten food sources supplying protein. I was getting a good amount of protein from these sources. I was also eating a lot of salad that included white beans, kidney beans and sometimes black beans, all good sources of protein. There's a dish that my wife makes with sautéed white beans, salmon and spinach that's outstanding. And I like almonds, another good source of protein. I was covered in the protein department.

A Healthy State

My brain had come through for me. I changed my diet and my eating habits in a relaxed fashion without any difficulty.

Getting my brain into a healthy, effectively functioning state was extremely important to me. Learning about the effects of oxidation and the foods that I needed to eat and drink, which included water, was making a major difference. The brain only knows what the brain knows, and I was learning a lot about what I needed to do to get my brain healthy again.

What I hadn't thought about is that when your brain is in trouble you don't have any pain, and it doesn't shout-out to let you know that it's in trouble. It just doesn't function as well.

The Law of Neuroplasticity is always changing the internal structure of your brain, laying down new pathways, moving those that aren't used as much to the back and "pruning" away those that aren't needed. It does this based on what you do or don't do. But whether you realize it or not your brain changes what you will do or won't do according to what it can and can't do.

In my case, the functioning ability of my brain had been negatively affected by what I was eating and drinking. It wasn't that I was excessively heavy or that the foods that I was eating were so horrendously bad. It was just that I was not eating or drinking what my brain needed to retain its health and good functioning ability. Now my brain was regaining its health and its functioning ability.

It wasn't that I was smarter. I am who I am and I'll always be that person. It was just that my brain was much more capable of doing things. That meant that I was much more capable, and it was opening up an entirely new, exciting world to me. My life was changing, and I wasn't going to let that go. But I wasn't finished yet.

Wanting to tell Everyone

At first I was really proud of myself. I knew all of this good stuff about the brain and the role that eating played in damaging it or keeping it healthy. I wanted everyone to know what I knew. I wanted everyone to do what I was planning to do because what I was doing was the right thing to do. I felt that what I knew gave me the right to tell people how bad the foods that they were eating were for the functioning of their brain.

Let me tell you, that doesn't go over very well. My wife kept telling me, but I only insisted that I was trying to help. They needed to know, and I arrogantly assumed that they wanted to know. It didn't take long before my wife and I stopped getting dinner invitations from our friends, and no one, it appeared, wanted to have lunch with me.

Once again, my wife was right. So, I turned to my kids. They would understand. Even follow my lead. Some of it rubbed off, but for the most part that didn't work. They're all grown with kids of their own. They have doctors for themselves and doctors for their children. They don't want a parent telling them what to eat. You can't explain everything you know about food and health to them. I've tried.

When you bull ahead like that you're really looking for justification. You're trying to make yourself feel good, but you end up making yourself feel like an outsider looking in. So if you're smart you back off.

I learned. I stopped talking about the brain and healthy eating when we went out unless asked, and no one ever asked. Our friends started asking us to go to dinner with them again, and I was able to make luncheon dates. I realized that the best you can do with your kids is to ask them to accommodate your eating habits when you visit. You can even ask good friends, but that's as far as it goes.

If they ask you why you will or won't eat certain things tell them, but make it brief.

You need to understand what you need to do and why, and you need to do it. If you want to talk about it with others you have to pick the right time and place. Otherwise you'll just end up on the outside looking in. You won't like that and you probably won't make the change.

Section Four - The Other Elements in the

Brain's Support System

Physical Activity and the Brain

By this time it was clear that there is no silver bullet when it comes to the brain. The brain is a system with pieces and parts that have evolved over the years with each having a purpose. Keeping your brain healthy and functioning effectively is really a matter of keeping the pieces and parts healthy so that they can do their job. It was in the late 90's when Dr. Elizabeth Gould proved that the hippocampus in the human brain produces new brain cells throughout life, albeit at different rates. The rate at which those cells are produced depends on what the individual is doing or not doing and the environment in which it's done. That led to the conclusion that the human brain is constantly changing based on what an individual is learning or not learning, what new information is being processed or not being processed. That makes the hippocampus the piece in the brain primarily responsible for memory and learning and an important part of my cognitive functioning.

The hippocampus generates new cells that are used to receive, process and retain new (experience-dependent) information. New brain cells either strengthen an existing functional network of cells or they join with other cells to create a new functional network. When functional networks are strengthened or new ones created the brain reorganizes its internal structure to accommodate them. If a cell is not used fairly quickly it will die off.

I understood the function of the hippocampus long before I learned what needed to be done to keep it healthy and functioning effectively. I knew that I had to keep learning, and I had to continue doing all the good things that I was doing. Then it appeared "*stress*".

Stress is a major factor in the health and functioning of the hippocampus.

What we refer to as "stress" initially functioned as the brain's early survival mechanism, and it still is. When the brain is alerted to danger it initiates the stress response. First it releases cortisol. Cortisol is a hormone that focuses the available resources needed to avoid or fight off the stressor. In addition to focusing resources cortisol holds back those parts of the system that aren't needed to deal with the stressor. Next, the brain brings extra energy to the stressed area in the form of adrenaline, a good, short term sugar substitute.

Unfortunately, when stress continues for too long the adrenaline dissipates. The cortisol hangs around continuing to function, but there's a change. Without it's sister hormone, adrenaline, cortisol becomes a highly toxic substance damaging and killing brain tissue, but the damage doesn't end there.

When the stress hormone cortisol is present resources are focused on the stressor. New brain cells processing new information become a distraction. Fewer cells are needed so fewer cells are produced. That causes the hippocampal areas to shrink in size. The reduction in size further limits the ability of the hippocampus to produce cells causing further shrinkage and the production of fewer cells. As you can imagine this has a negative affect on memory and learning. As it turns out physical exercise is a great way to relieve stress, and that makes good sense.

Fortunately, we've been physically active throughout our history, which goes back at least 40 million years. We needed to be physically active to survive. That's how the brain lived, and it still lives that way. When we're physically active we're doing something good. We have either escaped predators, obtained food, learned something new to help us survive, or possibly found a mate. All of that is good, and your brain responds to it.

The generation of new brain cells, along with the health of older cells, is dependent on an internally generated chemicals referred to as "*Brain Derived Neuronal Growth Factor*" (BDNGF). The first thing I thought of when I learned about BDNGF was Miracle Grow for plants. Overtly they function in much the same way. The difference is that the generation of BDNGF is very responsive to physical activity. The more physical activity the more BDNGF is produced, but it works the other way as well. Physical activity is more than just a stress reliever and generator of cell growth factors (BDNGF).

Typically, physical activity declines with age, and I was no different. I moved around a fair amount, but like most people today I spent a lot of time in front of a computer, and at night I didn't want to do anything. Needless to say I wasn't very physically active. I didn't consider myself to be a couch potato, but I wasn't very physically active and I didn't exercise.

I had belonged to a variety of gyms and health clubs throughout the years, but that always ended the same way. Since I didn't go to them regularly membership seemed to be a waste of money. I would let my membership lapse. But I still had that nagging feeling. I didn't know why, but I knew that I needed to exercise. My next step was to get some equipment for use at home.

The first piece of equipment I bought was a StairMaster. I started out with good intentions, but it just became a place to hang clothes. I ultimately got rid of it. Next was a combination treadmill and StairMaster. It was light and easy to move so I put it against a wall away from my closet. That way I couldn't hang clothes on it. The hybrid treadmill-stairmaster sat in my bedroom for about three years without being used. I didn't hang clothes on it, but the machine just stood there a constant reminder of what I needed to do. Then I started to learn about my brain.

It wasn't until 2008 that I read the newly published book "Sparks, The Revolutionary New Science of Exercise and the Brain" by John Ratey M.D. The book didn't discuss the effects of exercise on the various parts of the brain. It didn't even go into any detail about what affect exercise had on the body, but it did show that physical activity had a positive affect on memory and learning in school children. It didn't take long before the need to be physically active became widely recognized as a crucial element in supporting brain health and learning at all ages.

With all that I was doing my brain was going to be a lot healthier. But I knew that if I wanted to keep it healthy and take it's functioning to another level I needed to be more physically active.

Being physically active and regularly engaging in physical exercise would keep my blood vessels flexible, and healthy. My blood vessels could stretch and expand so that they could carry a greater volume of blood, along with its cargo, to my brain. But it didn't stop there.

Physical activity would increase the rate at which blood would flow to my brain. Blood feeds functioning brain cells by bringing the oxygen, water, nutrients and salts brain cells need to function. By increasing the rate at which the blood was flowing more of those things would get to my brain faster. My brain cells would be stimulated and function at a higher level. I would accomplish more.

Dopamine is the neurotransmitter of memory and learning. Dopamine is also the reward neurotransmitter which is why being physically active makes you feel good. In addition to making you feel good an increase in dopamine production will increase focus, memory and the ability to learn.

There were other major benefits of physical activity. By increasing the flow of blood to the brain cells are hydrated, inflammation is reduced, material for needed repair and rebuilding are provided, enzymes are activated, signals between cells are strengthened, and new tissue is built.

All of this was enough to convince me that staying physically active was important to the health and functioning of my brain. I was convinced. It was the next step I had to take.

Initially, I had accepted the fact that I needed to exercise. But I had only accepted it intellectually. I knew I had to do it so I did it. But, like eating, my Emotional Sub-brain was still hung up on my old habits. It wasn't going to make this change overnight, and it certainly wasn't going to make it easy.

I started using my hybrid-treadmill first thing in the morning before I showered. At first, exercising was a novelty. "…I'm actually exercising. How neat!…" I was proud of it, but like my experience with the gyms it became drudgery. I even found myself staying in bed longer just to avoid it. You know the old excuse. "…I'm tired… I don't have the time…I'll do it tomorrow…" This time there was a difference.

My brain was involved, and my brain knew that we had to exercise. When you engage in aerobic exercise with some regularity your brain begins to expect it. Now, if I missed exercising on my treadmill-stairmaster or walking I didn't feel as good. My brain was in the act, and if I didn't exercise it made me feel like I had committed a crime. Even with that exercising was not easy. It was work.

I'm not sure when or why the change came about. There wasn't an identifiable seam. Maybe it was when Diane suggested alternating my morning workouts with long walks, and that's what we did. Not only were we getting good physical exercise, but it gave us time to just be together. Now, I'll frequently do both.

I felt good, but I felt much better and much sharper when I exercised regularly. My brain was up there goading me on, and like water, exercising just became a part of who I am. More importantly it became a part of who I wanted to be.

Why do we Need to Sleep?

Have you ever asked yourself why you need to sleep? You know that if you don't get enough sleep you're tired. Sometimes if you get too much sleep you get tired as well. You know that when you're tired you're not usually as sharp as you would like. It's a little more difficult for you to focus and concentrate on things. Your memory isn't as swift as it normally is, and your reasoning ability probably declines. There's one thing more.

Most of us have experienced being tired and trying to reason something out, or solve a problem, possibly work a puzzle. We're stumped. No matter how hard we try it alludes us. Then in the morning after a good nights rest we wake up and what we were having difficulty with the night before becomes perfectly clear. That tells you that something happened during your sleeping hours that allowed your brain to receive and interpret information more clearly than it did when you were tired. You were able to focus, interpret and reason. Not to make a pun, but that's pretty "heady".

Like most other people I just accepted "sleep" as something that I had to do. It was necessary. When I was a young child I was told that I needed to sleep, but no one ever told me why. It was ingrained in me, as I'm sure it was in you, that you needed sleep. Sleep is good for you. Everyone seems to know that we needed sleep. Part of that is due to our ancient history which was responsive to light and dark.

If you go way, way, way back, maybe 40,000 years, when the first homo-sapiens were to have appeared they didn't have artificial light. All they had was the sun. All they knew was that when the sun was out they could see. When it was not out it was dark and they couldn't see.

The light made it easier to forage for food, hunt, and fight off predators. There was nothing that they could really do when it was dark so they slept. The development of fire was an improvement, but fire was stationary. It allowed for the cooking of food, but didn't really help with those other things. Then there was an advance in technology and the torch came along. That helped some with identifying and fighting off predators, but when it was dark it was dark, and there was not much to do so the people slept. They went to sleep early (by our standards), but they got up at daybreak. As a result, they got 10-12 hours of sleep each night.

The light, dark became a cycle that we adhered to, and that established our internal rhythms. To a great extent that rhythm is still with us. Unfortunately, that's not the end of it. Along came the torch, the gas lamp and the electric light. Now we could keep the light on all the time if we had sufficient fuel or sufficient money to pay the electric bill, but we still needed to sleep. That leaves us with the question "Why do we need to sleep?"

We have part of the answer. The light-dark rhythms of our Brainbody System push us in that direction, but that still begs the question "Why do we need to sleep and why does sleep help to replenish out cognitive abilities?"

Up until recently "sleep" and why we need it have remained a mystery. There is still no comprehensive answer that would satisfy all of the questions, but we have a lot of answers and we keep getting more.

Reflect on your own behavior for a moment. When you're tired you can't work as well. You're learning, judgment, reasoning, and problem solving abilities are impaired. Your reflexes are even slowed down.

Reflexes are controlled by signals sent from your nerves to your brain and back again to activate an action by a muscle. Reflexes occur as a result of your brain responding to and processing physical information. Without the appropriate amount of sleep your brain doesn't process or respond to information as rapidly.

Your brain works 24 hours a day receiving, interpreting, prioritizing, processing and storing information, deciding on actions to be taken, determining where and how to take them, and sending the appropriate messages to the appropriate places. That's a lot of work.

Your brain is even working when you're sleeping, but what's it doing? What happens when you're sleeping?

First, you're in a very defined area which means that your skin is only able to sense and transmit a limited amount of information most of which is repetitive. Second, your eyes are closed so visual information is shut down. Third, your ears are receiving the same or no sound, which means that your brain doesn't have to pay close attention to the information coming from your auditory nerves. Your brain is alert, though, to any changes. If there's an unusual sound, an extremely loud noise, or something that your brain feels might indicate danger, it will wake you.

Fourth, the external elements such as your arms, legs, and other body muscles don't have to work. They don't need help and direction from your brain. That allows your brain to concentrate on its own tasks. Sleep sets the stage for your brain to work uninterrupted, but your brain goes one step further. It slows down your breathing along with other system functions, and focuses the use of your blood on its needs to gain maximum advantage from its contents. Now, you're asleep. You have been shut down, or slowed way down, so that your brain can work. What does it do while you're sleeping?

I don't know in what order it does these things. Perhaps no one knows, but there are a number of things that your brain has to do so that it can continue to function effectively. Your brain has been receiving information, both internally and externally, all of the time you've been awake. It has acted on some of that information, but it has to create permanent memories and connections for most or all of it while eliminating that information that has no relevance or priority. Additionally, it has to clear the information that's in the system so that it's prepared to receive and process new information. That could mean accumulating similar information that relates to a problem, as well as solving the problem.

To begin with, sleep is the brain's administrative and housekeeping period. I'm sure that at one time or another you've tried to do something over the phone, possibly even on the computer and experienced "Sorry, the computer is down at this time for maintenance … We should be available again for consumer support in (hours) …". It seems most likely, that if your brain is your control center it's shutting you down for maintenance by having you sleep.

The next thing requires a little insight. I've said it before, your brain is not like an arm or a leg or an organ in your body that is hurting. When those things are hurting you know about it, but when it comes to the brain you don't have a clue. Yet, brain tissue, and along with it the cells it carries, are constantly being damaged and depleted due to toxins, use and time. New tissue needs to be built. Damaged and depleted tissue has to be repaired and rebuilt.

For your brain to function and support your cognitive abilities it needs time for maintenance and administration. It wants to get back into shape and it needs to get back into shape for you to continue to process new information and survive. Most adults require 7-10 hours of sleep to allow their brain to accomplish these tasks. Now you know "Why we need sleep?", and if anyone asks you can tell them.

Your Blood and Blood Delivery System

BLOOD

Until all of this happened to me I never really thought much about my blood. That was something for my doctor to look at and worry about. I had to have a blood test once a year, but as far as I knew it was OK. The truth is that I never really understood the relationship between my blood and my brain. My blood was there just like my brain, and I knew that without it I wouldn't live, but that was about as far as it went.

Once I started to study those things that had an impact on how the brain functioned it became obvious that blood was a key player. Your brain can't function without blood. I knew that. Everyone knows that. What I didn't understand was that the blood that was circulating through my brain played a major role in how it functioned and that had a major impact on how I how I functioned cognitively.

The more new information that we receive and process the more cognitively-able we become. The brain only knows what it knows and the more it knows about its environment the greater the possibility of surviving. We have brain cells organized in functional networks to accomplish that. There's no rest for your brain cells and cell networks. They work 24 hours a day, 7 days a week, even when you're sleeping. Those cells are busy receiving, processing, interpreting, sorting deciding, directing, signaling, building, repairing and getting the things done that need to be done. How well they perform each of those tasks is dependent on their health and what they are able to do

As humans we would have trouble competing in a natural environment. We are not particularly strong. We're not fast. Our skin is not particularly protective and we have a relatively poor sense of smell. We are susceptible to the elements and there are limits to the temperature range in which we can exist. We survive because of our cognitive abilities. Those abilities depend on the health and functioning ability of our brain cells.

Each cell has a job to do, a function to perform. Typically one-third of all neurons (brain cells) support cognitive functioning. But in order for a brain cell to live it must be supported by a supply of blood. That seems simple enough except that your brain is very particular about where it distributes its blood. For a cell to be supported with blood it must belong to a functional network of cells. Each functional network of cells has a common task to perform. Each cell performs a function so that as a whole the network of cells fulfills that task. For a cell to do its job it needs to be receiving a continuous supply of blood. More accurately, it needs to receive what's in that blood.

I was losing cognitive abilities one at a time. What I didn't realize was that it wasn't happening to me for no reason. I was allowing it to happen. I didn't realize it but I was constantly generating and killing off brain cells depending on what I did or didn't do. And I wasn't using my blood to keep my brain cells healthy and functioning effectively.

Your brain is your control center. As your control center it controls everything in, and on, the Brain-body System. It even controls what you think and what you do. To accomplish that your brain has approximately100 billion living, functioning, cells, neurons, organized into functional networks having approximately one- hundred trillion connections with approximately one-third of them responsible for cognitive functioning. Your Logical Executive Sub-brain, with its cognitive tools, needs to draw a lot of blood to stay healthy and function effectively.

To remain healthy and do their jobs effectively your brain cells need uncontaminated oxygen, clean water, anti-oxidants to defend against oxidative damage, omega polyunsaturated fats to build tissue, protein as workers and complex carbohydrates to provide it with energy.

If any of these things are missing, or under provided, the health of your cells and cellular networks will deteriorate. The cells won't be able to do the same job they did when they were healthy. They will become less and less productive. Eventually they will draw less and less blood, become dysfunctional and die. As that's happening your capabilities, probably your cognitive capabilities, will be affected.

That's what had been happening to me. In addition to teaching my brain how not to function so that I could speak, I hadn't been providing it with the things that it needed to stay healthy and function effectively. I didn't know that my brain was telling me anything by how it was performing, but I was wrong.

The brain is not like an arm or leg or any organ in or on your body. If something is wrong with one of those you feel it. Most likely you experience pain. That doesn't happen with the brain. It has no pain nerves. The only way that you can tell that your brain is not healthy is in its lack of performance.

When your brain is hurting your cognitive abilities won't function as well. Memory keeps getting worse. Learning, problem solving, and reasoning get much more difficult. Eventually, even physical function is affected. As I learned, when this happens the world in which you live becomes smaller and smaller and how you perceive it becomes narrower and narrower.

What does this all have to do with blood? It's your blood that carries the oxygen, the water, anti-oxidants, unsaturated fats, protein, complex carbohydrates and ionized salts to your brain. Your blood is a carrier of freight like UPS, Roadway or Yellow Freight. With freight carriers it's the packages in the truck awaiting delivery that are important. It's the same thing with blood.

Oxygen, water, nutrients and ionized salts are the packages that your blood carries and delivers to your brain. If the right packages are delivered in the right quantities at the right time your brain will stay healthy and work effectively. I was responsible for what was going into my blood for delivery to my brain and I hadn't been doing a good job. Once I understood that I knew what I had to do.

You can visualize a stream of blood as having three segments; blood plasma, red cells and white cells. Blood plasma is responsible for carrying the water, nutrients and ionized salts that your brain needs to function. Red blood cells are iron rich and responsible for carrying oxygen. They also attract and carry carbon dioxide to your lungs so that it can be eliminated. White blood cells are like the Marines aboard ship. The circulating blood carries them to points of attack where they are deployed to fight infection or trauma.

For your brain to function at its best it needs uncontaminated oxygen, sufficient amounts of water to stay fully hydrated, and the right nutrients. Anything less and the health and functioning of your brain will suffer. You probably won't realize it until you get to the point where you feel that age has started to do you in. But it's not age. I learned that. I was responsible for loading all of the right things into my blood, and I hadn't done a very good job.

If my brain is my control center, and I am responsible for loading all of the things that are needed into my blood, it stands to reason that it was my brain that messed up. That's true, but that's not the complete picture. My brain only knew what it knew. It didn't know any more. I had never associated any of these things with the health and functioning of my brain. What was worse was all of the bad information that my brain was receiving from the environment where I lived, worked and played; supermarkets with all of their processed and fatty foods, sugary drinks and simple carbs, fast food outlets with more fatty foods and sugary drinks, and TV ads encouraging me to eat all the wrong things. That's what my brain knew at the time. It knew what was easily available, and that was a big part of my problem. But I was learning. My brain was receiving new information. This time it was receiving the correct information and it was responding to it.

There's more to blood than just understanding what it carries to your brain. Your blood can change with time, and circumstances. The thickness of your blood, its volume and its delivery speed can change based on how much water you drink, how physically active you are, the temperature of your environment and the amount of stress you're under.

Blood circulation is altered when you're sleeping so that more blood goes to your brain, and less to those parts of your body that aren't in use. If there's a stressor your brain will direct more blood, with its contents, to the area fighting off the stressor. And, of course, the content of your blood is altered depending on what you've eaten or had to drink.

The fact that your brain consumes 20-25% of the cargo in your blood suggests that it's also producing 20-25% of the total waste produced by your System. If that waste isn't removed your brain function will slow down to a crawl. It's the water in your blood that removes that waste. After it delivers its load, your blood removes the potentially toxic debris, like oxidants and dead cells, from your brain and carry's it to those places where it can be eliminated from your system.

Because of the essential elements that it delivers and removes blood is critical to the functioning and survival of your brain. That makes blood your brains primary resource. Like any other living thing dependent on a resource for survival it wants to conserve as much of it as possible. The Law of Neuroplasticity takes care of that problem for your brain.

The Law of Neuroplasticity is constantly rearranging your brain cells, cell networks and their connections. It does this for two key reasons both of which are related to the use of blood. First, it kills off new and old cells that aren't being used by depriving them of blood. Second, it rearranges functioning cells to ensure effective communication between active cells with a minimum of blood use. Overall the Law of Neuroplasticity is ensuring that blood, the brain's primary resource, is used efficiently.

I didn't know any of this. What an eye opener! What was really enlightening was the fact that the health and functioning of my brain were dependent on what was delivered in my blood, and that I was responsible for the cargo that went into my blood.

YOUR BLOOD DELIVERY SYSTEM

Your blood is a big, constantly working, transport system carrying essential cargo to your brain. If you consider the fact that trucks require roads along which to travel, and trains require tracks, then it stands to reason that blood would need some type of path to travel along as well. It also stands to reason that the condition of these paths would play an important role in the ease, speed and quantity of the blood that can travel on them. That's where your Blood Delivery System comes in.

Your doctor probably refers to your blood delivery system as your circulatory system. I found that name to be too academic, and removed from what it really does. So, for my purposes, I called the circulatory system the Blood Delivery System. That's what it does. The Blood Delivery System allows blood to deliver its cargo throughout the Brain-body System. But, your brain is its biggest and most important customer using 20-25% of your blood along with it's contents.

Your Blood Delivery System is what you would expect it to be, your blood vessels, heart and lungs. Your blood vessels are your arteries, capillaries and veins, but your blood would deplete, be dirty and lay dormant in those vessels if it wasn't for your heart and lungs.

Your heart and lungs are the engines that receive, clean and drive the blood through your system.

Your heart is like a responsible and conscientious traffic cop. It wants everything moving in the right direction at the right time and to the right place without disruption. It also wants to make sure that it doesn't get clean blood and used blood mixed up so it separates them.

The heart receives and redirects clean blood on one side through a network of major and minor arteries and capillaries. The other side of the heart receives and redirects used blood with its waste and toxins

Arteries and capillaries only receive and carry "clean" blood. The clean blood includes the new blood and contains the oxygen, water and nutrients. Used blood is carried in the veins and contains waste and toxins that have been gathered for elimination.

Arteries can be likened to highways. There are major highways like interstates that carry you to regional areas. There are secondary or smaller highways within each of those areas that take you to specific locations. In this case the secondary highways are smaller arteries carrying clean blood, with its cargo, back to local distribution points. Capillaries pick up the new blood at the local distribution points and transport it back to the cells that it serves.

Because capillaries are very narrow and have thin walls they can only carry small quantities of blood. For a cell to function it must receive blood from its capillary, but that works two ways. The quantity of blood and the speed with which its delivered will depend on the need of the cells, the condition of the capillaries, and the rate at which the heart and lungs are pumping.

Capillaries supply blood to functioning cells. If cells are not active the amount of blood going through its capillary will decline. That can become a problem. Unlike arteries the walls of a capillary are thin, and are typically supported against collapse by the blood flowing through them.

If the amount of blood going through the capillary declines its walls can start to sag. If blood flow continues to decline the walls of the capillary will eventually collapse cutting off blood flow completely, killing the brain cells on the route and diminishing or eliminating some type of function, possibly a cognitive function. If one or more cells in a network aren't functioning, as may occur in a stroke or head trauma, it affects the overall capability of the functioning network of cells.

Although your brain weighs under 3lbs. and accounts for less than 2% of your body weight it uses 20 – 25% of your blood along with its contents. That makes the amount of new blood delivered to your brain extremely important to its health and functioning. That makes the health and ability of blood vessels to carry blood a critical part of brain health.

That brings us to the third type of blood vessel, the vein. "Vein" is a term used colloquially to refer to all blood vessels, but that's far from accurate. Arteries and capillaries carry new blood to major and regional areas. Capillary's carry blood to local customers where the oxygen, water and nutrients that it brings are used. That usage produces waste and toxins in the form of oxidants. It's the veins that carry away the blood after its been used.

Lungs can be thought of as a strong, highly complex pump with a mission. Lungs clean and replenish the blood that it receives by getting rid of the carbon dioxide and other toxic gases while at the same time bringing in a fresh supply of oxygen.

The in-out pumping action of your lungs takes place when you breathe. It's the rate of your breathing that determines the rate at which your lungs pump blood. Your level of physical activity will affect the rate at which you breath. Carrying that further, it's the in-out pumping action of your lungs that determines the rate at which your blood is cleaned, replenished, sent back to your heart and redistributed to those points where it's needed. The rate at which your lungs are pumping will determine how quickly cargo can be delivered and used by your brain. The condition of your heart and blood vessels will determine how fast and how much cargo can be delivered.

Blood vessels aren't inert like walls of a pipe. They're made up of millions, possibly billions, of living, functioning, actively working, cells. Like any other cell they require oxygen, water, glucose, nutrients, vitamins and minerals to function. Arteries have relatively thick tissue which is comprised of millions of cells. These cells have their own capillaries supplying blood and cargo.

Your brain has a constant requirement for blood, even when you're sleeping. Actually, your brain normally uses more blood when you're sleeping then when you're awake. The amount of blood that your brain receives when you're awake or asleep will in part be determined by the health of your Blood Delivery System.

Any plaque, blockages or leaks in your blood vessels will reduce the amount of blood going to your brain. Blood vessels containing plaque, narrow, become stiff and frequently crack. Wall cells don't function as well or at all reducing the supply of blood they can carry. Even if you don't actually have a stroke your brain function will be affected, possibly your cognitive functioning. That makes the health of your Blood Delivery System incredibly important to the health and functioning of your brain.

Section Five - A Brain Healthy Life Style

Moving into a Brain Healthy Life

I've presented the Functioning Brain as being comprised of a Primary brain and two assistants, the Emotional Sub-brain and the Logical Executive sub-brain. I've said that the internal structure of your brain is controlled by the laws of neurogenesis and neuroplasticity, that those laws are responsive to what you do or don't do, that your brain functions according to certain rules, that your brain must continue to process new information throughout your life, that you need to continue to learn, that your ability to process information and learn is dependent on the health of your brain, and that the functioning and cognitive health of your brain are dependent on the support that you provide. That includes staying hydrated, eating the right foods, being physically active, getting an appropriate amount of sleep and minimizing long term stress.

It sounds like there's a lot you have to do, and there probably is, but you shouldn't feel that moving into a brain healthy life is a sacrifice that you have to make to keep age from robbing you of your cognitive abilities. Quite the contrary. Moving into a brain healthy life style will take you into an exciting new world. A world where you learn new things, become more physically and socially active and feel sharper.

EVERYONE IS DIFFERENT
Everyone is different. Everyone has different habits, different interests. Some of you are physically active, some not, and some of you are in between. You have different diets, different eating habits, and some of you may be learning new things and some not. The only thing I can assume is that if you've read this book you're interested in having a healthy, effectively functioning brain. How you move into a brain healthy life style is up to you. It will be different for everyone, but there is a path you can follow.

To start with, look at the content of your life. What are you doing? When I started writing this book I was focused on people 50+, but the more I got into it, and the more research I did, the more I realized that brain health, particularly cognitive health, should be everyone's concern at every age. It's just that those of us that are over 50 have been subjected to the overbearing influence of a myth. That myth has everyone believing that aging causes cognitive decline.

YOUR PHYSICAL SELF

A brain healthy life style has to start with you, your physical condition, your health and how physically active you are or are not. You need your information gathering and processing equipment to be in good shape in order to stay cognitively healthy. That starts with information gathering. Vision and hearing are your two primary information gathering sensors. The first thing that you want to do is to evaluate their functioning effectiveness. How well are you seeing and hearing?

If your vision or hearing sensors are not functioning properly you are not receiving complete or accurate information. That will affect your cognitive functioning. Vision or hearing problems will affect "*focus*" and "*focus*" is a major element of "*memory*". If you have hearing or vision problems, there's a good chance that you're missing some of the things that are going on around you (your environment). The problem may be minor at first and what you're missing might not make much of a difference, but there's a good chance it will get worse. You've adapted to the problem at its early stages so it's probable that you'll just adapt to the increasing difficulty it presents without realizing it. Talk to the people around you. They'll know. If you have hearing or vision problems, regardless of age, they need to be *fixed*.

The next thing that you need to do is to address any health problems that you might have. General health problems can affect your memory and cognitive functioning without your realizing it. It's important to find out whether your blood pressure is within acceptable norms, if your red blood cell count is low, do you have chronically high blood sugar, does your thyroid function normally, is there a reason to believe that you may possibly have Lyme disease? What about medications that you take? For example, statins have been known to produce dementia like symptoms in some people. Any of these can affect your cognitive functioning. Get checked out by a doctor. It may just be a routine visit, but it might also save you from some serious cognitive problems.

BEING PHYSICALY ACTIVE
To be brain healthy you need to be physically active. Physical activity is needed for the production of new brain cells. Physical activity helps to keep your blood vessels soft and flexible, increases blood flow to the brain, stimulates the production of glutathione, the brain's super anti-oxidant, and helps generate new, experience-dependent brain cells. Being physically active increases your production of dopamine. Dopamine is the memory and learning neurotransmitter. Good dopamine levels are needed to process, remember and use newly processed information. Increased dopamine levels also helps increase incentive, mood and outlook. Being physically active is essential for a brain healthy life. Being physically active doesn't mean just exercising.

If you can't be physically active because of work make accommodations. It will help your brain and your work. If you're in front of a computer most of the day, take breaks about every hour even if it's just to walk down the hall to get a drink of water. You also have to make sure that you get, at least, one-half hour of continuous physical exercise a day. It could just be walking briskly. Sauntering doesn't count. If you're going to exercise the best times are first thing in the morning or mid-day.

If you're not walking briskly, or reasonably long distances, because you become short of breath then you need to see a doctor. Being able to breath properly in response to physical activity is a major element of good brain health. Your lungs are part of your brain's Blood Delivery System. If they're not functioning as they should it will affect your cognitive health and eventually your cognitive functioning.

Make it fun! Try walking, dancing, swimming, hiking, biking, or anything else that interests you and that will keep you physically active. Try something that you haven't tried before like yoga, pilates, kick boxing, basketball, hockey, skating. Just make sure that you're physically able to do those things that you attempt. Even if you think that your age prevents you from doing something that you want to do, I'll bet that there's a group somewhere that will fit your needs and that you can join. Search for it.

If you have physical disabilities that limit your physical activity don't give up. Talk to your doctor. Identify those things that can help with vascular flexibility and blood flow, and the ones that you can do. It might be difficult at first but the effort will pay off.

YOUR LIFE CONTENT
Next, look at the content of your life. What are you doing? Are you working all the time? Are you out and about? Are you involved in something outside of yourself? Are you meeting people? Do you consider yourself an active part of your community? Or is everyday pretty much the same?

Can you say that you're learning? Learning means that you're processing new information. If you want to maintain brain health and good cognitive function you need to keep learning. That means new things. Processing the same information with different names won't work. Being socially active and involved is a form of learning and processing new information, but so is learning a new skill. Even if you can only spend fifteen minutes a day learning a new skill it's important to your cognitive health.

If you're working you have time constraints. You're probably tired when you get home. It's easy to do nothing, but it's a cognitive downer. Find something that you would like to do or learn, either by yourself or with a group, AND DO IT. Even if it only means spending 15 to 30 minutes in the evening on it. Persistence is critical to getting into a brain healthy life, and it's worth every minute.

There are plenty of things out there just waiting for you, even reading a book. There's a good chance you don't even have to go outside. I doubt that playing a video game would qualify unless you don't play video games as a rule. The important thing is that you do something different for yourself. Challenge your brain to do and learn something new. As a suggestion you can learn to play a musical instrument or to square dance. You can probably think of other things but you need to be active and involved, and above all you need to have fun doing it.

It's tough to get going, but the more you do the more you'll do, and the less you do the less you'll do. If you want to keep your cognitive brain healthy you have to keep doing.

HYDRATION
While you're involved in being physically and socially active start drinking water. Don't stress yourself worrying about how much water you should drink. You don't want to make getting into a brain healthy life style an onerous task. Relax! Do what you can do as you can do it, but be conscious of what it is you need to do.

Your urine plays an important role in brain health by removing waste and toxins from your Brain-body System. That means that you have a hydration indicator with you at all times; your urine. Ideally, your urine should be clear with very little color.

Don't go out and in one day try to become fully hydrated. It won't work. A combination of things will actually determine the color of your urine and your level of hydration. That's going to be a little different for everyone, and it's going to change from day to day, probably within each day. The important thing is that you know where you are with hydration and based on that what to do about it.

Where you are, what you're doing, what you're eating and drinking, the amount and quality of sleep you got the night before, the level of stress you're under, even the weather, can influence your level of hydration along with the color of your urine. Don't worry about hour by hour changes. You'll go nuts and won't accomplish anything.

Monitor the color of your urine. You want each day to show a little improvement. You know that you can lighten your urine by drinking more water, eating more fruits and vegetables or drinking milk. Vegetable juice and cocoa work as well. They're good sources of water, but just plain water is the best.

Based on the color of your urine when you start you're going to take a stab at how much more water you need circulating in your system. It's going to be trial and error so take your best guess as a way to get started. I've said that everyone is different, and that's obviously true, but there are certain consistencies.

Your brain has been working all night using water. You need water first thing in the morning. Drink water after you've exercised or done something strenuous. You will need water during and after a lot of heavy brain work. Drink water when you've been sweating. You need more water when it's hot out. Don't let yourself get thirsty. If you are thirsty your Brain-body System is already starting to crave water and that includes your brain.

Fruit juices and soda aren't brain healthy. In fact, most fruit juices, particularly those you buy, have little nutrient benefit and lots of sugar. Until you get the color of your urine under control stick with water, milk, cocoa or vegetable juice as your drinks of choice.

Caffeine is a diuretic, but if you're drinking coffee or tea you're adding water as well so it probably balances out. It's really more a question of how much caffeine you can consume before it becomes detrimental. The general consensus is that two to three cups of tea or coffee a day shouldn't be damaging. If you need a hot beverage in the morning try decaf coffee, green tea or hot chocolate. If you need sugar add it yourself. Tea has half of the caffeine that coffee has and green tea is loaded with anti-oxidants. Remember, drinks with caffeine don't add water. Whatever beverage you select try to drink it without adding sugar.

There's been a lot of conversation around caffeine. Some studies have concluded that caffeine is good for memory, some say it's not. The general consensus is that caffeine has short term affects as a stimulant for memory, but has no lasting effect and can prove to be harmful. Limit your intake of caffeine.

STOP THE DAMAGE DOING
I can't say it enough. You don't want this to be a Herculean struggle. You don't want to stress-out about having to do this or that. You want to move into your new brain healthy life style easily. Unfortunately, there is one area that might present a problem going this route. Sugar!

Sugar is contained in the foods you eat. You've been consuming sugar in some form or another since you were first born. The foods that contained the sugar you've been ingesting were either a complex sugar (complex carbohydrate) or a simple sugar (simple carbohydrate). That seems easy enough. But sugar is a sneaky, feel good food.

Sugar is the oldest source of energy for the brain. That makes it a survival food. Over the millions of years that have gone by your brain has become extra sensitive to sugar. It craves sugar. After all, sugar means energy. Energy means survival, and your brain wants to survive. That allows sugar to come in the disguise of a friend and stay on as an enemy. Sugar convinces you that it's good. You like sugar and you like the foods that contain sugar.

Until the last seventy-five years or so most of the sugar we consumed was in the form of a complex carbohydrate. But our culture has gotten very good at popularizing and making available the foods we really like; the foods we'll buy. Those are the foods that contain simple sugars. Unfortunately, sugar is like an opiate to the brain. The more sugar it gets the more sugar it wants. You become motivated to eat and drink more foods rich in sugar. You feel like you need to eat something. What you really need is more sugar, simple carbohydrates. When that craving for something sweet hits you be aware of the fact that it's not the food your brain wants it's the sugar.

If you ignore the impact of sugar on your brain you will have a problem. Your sugar intake will eventually overwhelm the anti-oxidant capability of your brain (glutathione) and possibly your insulin's ability to balance the sugar in your blood. Once sugar has a foothold it hangs around to oxidize and destroy tissue. That damages the functioning of brain cells, possibly cells you need for your cognitive abilities.

You can't live without sugar. Sugar enters your blood as glucose which is the brain's best source of energy. Your brain is constantly working, converting fuel (glucose) to energy and causing something to happen, even when you're asleep. What you do or don't do determines how much sugar (glucose) your brain needs, but your brain can't store fuel. It can't store anything. Your brain has to use the sugar it receives to a productive end or burn and waste it. There-in lies your potential problem.

When your brain converts fuel (sugar) to energy it produces waste whether the fuel has been burned for a productive use or not,. That waste takes the form of oxidants. Since your brain is constantly working your brain is constantly producing oxidants. If your brain's internal anti-oxidant, glutathione, doesn't get rid of those oxidants they will attack and damage tissue looking for a balancing electrical charge. That causes oxidation and oxidative damage. A buildup of oxidative damage is referred to as oxidative stress. Oxidative stress has been identified as a primary cause of cognitive decline in aging.

Historically, your brain will need and receive 20-25% of the available sugar for fuel. That suggests that your brain will produce 20-25% of the waste that occurs from converting sugar to energy. Since your brain can't store fuel you want it to receive just the right amount of fuel it needs to do the work its doing. Any more than that will be burned creating unnecessary toxic waste.

Your brain is very forgiving. You can repair the damage that's been done, but if you want a healthy effectively functioning brain you have to stop damaging the cells. You have to stop the damage doing. Sugar is only your friend if you don't overdo it and it can be metabolized and burned gradually. Simple sugars are not your friend. Simple sugars are the primary damage-doers. Try to keep your intake to an absolute minimum.

An easy way to start is by changing white bread for whole grain bread, white rice for brown rice, or wild rice. If you're adventurous use quinoa. Try whole grain pastas. They're good and they're good for you. A baked russet potato works and so do sweet potatoes.

The next step is going to be more difficult. You will need to get rid of the sugary drinks (soda and fruit juice), the candy, the pastry, and the sugary cereals. I would guess that you probably want to stop reading at this point. By now though, you should realize that it's the sugar that's talking not your Logical Executive Sub-brain.

In essence, you will be taking yourself off of an opiate. You're going to need a *treat* for psychological and physical reasons. That treat will be in some form of sugar. Establish a *"treat time"* of the day and select something that you really like but limits your sugar intake. It may take a few weeks, but your brain will get used to it and start expecting its sugar treat at a certain time of the day.

There are some basic differences between simple and complex sugars. Simple sugars typically have little, if any, nutrient value whereas complex sugars usually have good nutrient value. The other differences between simple sugars and complex sugars is the speed and quantity with which they enter the blood. Simple sugars enter the blood quickly and are delivered en masse producing a large quantity of oxidants at one time. That overwhelms the brain's ability to counteract it. Eating an excessive amount of complex carbohydrates at one time will do the same thing. *Sugar is sugar!* If you're going to eat for brain health you have to minimize your intake of simple sugars. You also have to limit what you eat at one time.

To avoid excessive eating and provide your brain with fuel gradually, change the way you eat and drink water. Eat small amounts of food about every two and one-half hours. You don't need a meal every time you eat something. A piece of fruit, a glass of vegetable juice, a salad, a peanut butter and jelly sandwich, an open face turkey sandwich are examples of the kind of eating that works. I happen to like hummus with baby carrots, whole grain pita or flat bread. Just avoid eating the same thing throughout the day. You want to balance what you eat between complex carbs, protein, fruits and vegetables, unsaturated fats and, of course, you'll be drinking water.

Eating this way will allow your brain's internal defense force (glutathione) to do its job minimizing, or possibly eliminating, oxidant damage. That gives the healing, repair and building process a chance to work. You'll find that eating this way will reduce your overall intake of food. That reduction should produce a gradual drop in weight.

I stopped consuming any type of alcoholic beverage in the 80's. As a result, I have a personal bias. For that reason I have not dealt with beer or alcohol in this book, but you should know that they are simple sugars and constrict blood vessels reducing blood flow to the brain. That has a negative effect on cognitive ability.

I'm not a saint and I doubt that you are. I mess up every once and awhile as will you. That's not the end of the world and you shouldn't feel guilty about it as long as your mess-ups are controlled and limited. When you do mess-up don't just ignore it. Tell yourself that you've messed up, and get right back on track so that you can maintain your brain healthy life style, in this case your brain healthy eating habits.

I found a good website that will help you to identify and avoid simple sugars. And I'm passing the link on to you. www.wikihow. com/Avoid-Simple-Sugars. Also, I've explained simple sugars (carbohydrates) more extensively in the Appendix.

BUILDING YOUR DEFENSE FORCE

You've minimized your eating of simple sugars and you're eating small amounts of food throughout the day. You've given your internal anti-oxidant, glutathione, a chance at being successful, and you've taken a major step toward stopping the damage-doing. It would be a good idea at this point to increase your consumption of fruits and vegetables. Since fruits and vegetables are typically rich in anti-oxidants, they will build and reinforce your defense force. They will also help to offset some of that sugar loss from simple carbohydrates. I've found it particularly helpful to eat a piece of fruit when I have a craving for something. The craving was most likely caused by the need for sugar and the sugar in the fruit seems to satisfy the need.

Anti-oxidants are vitamins A, C and E. Oxidants are not all the same and are attracted to different anti-oxidants. You want to eat a variety of fruits and vegetables. I wouldn't get overly concerned about whether you should eat this or that to do this or that. Eat the fruits and vegetables that you enjoy. Eat the ones that are in your price range. Just don't stick to the same things all the time. Try to vary your selection. Frozen fruits and vegetables are almost as good as fresh. They're frequently more readily available and less expensive than the fresh variety.

To some extent the fruits and vegetables that you're able to obtain will be dependent on the season. You might also find that you can obtain a better selection of fruits and vegetables at a store other than the one where you normally shop. If you are not going to buy frozen try to get your fruits and vegetables so that they're relatively fresh. Most areas have supermarkets and farmer's markets that will provide you with what you need. Farmers markets are a great place to go but they're typically higher priced. "Fresh" fruits and vegetables provide taste that's difficult to find at the supermarket.

Begin building a habit of having a salad, or at least a green vegetable, with your primary meal of the day. In my case, that's usually dinner. Eat a small salad at other times during the day. They make a good snack. I try to keep a small bowl of grape tomatoes, sugar snap peas and baby carrots on my desk to snack on. You can try that or some other combination. Get rid of that hamburger, fries and soda at lunchtime (at any time) and replace it with a tasty salad perhaps with added chicken or tuna. But watch out. Select a salad dressing that's low in sugar something like a wine-vinaigrette.

You probably think that you're going to starve. I don't know where it came from but the term *bunny food* comes to mind. You're not trying to be a vegetarian or a vegan. You're just trying to eat so that your brain is healthy and can function effectively.

Remember, your brain is responsive to "What you do and don't do … It determines what you can and can't do … and what you will and won't do …" By keeping your brain healthy so that it can function more effectively you might be surprised at all the new things that you'll find yourself doing.

FOCUSING ON FAT

By now you're drinking water, having small amounts of food throughout the day, avoiding or minimizing simple sugars in your diet, and eating more fruits and vegetables. The next step in stopping the damage-doing is to focus on the type of fats that you need to consume.

The fats needed by your brain have to help reduce or eliminate tissue inflammation. Even if you've stopped the damage-doing from the foods your ingesting your brain tissues wear overtime. They gradually deplete. That causes tissue inflammation. Then there's the cortisol toxin from stress, and there may possibly be other toxins that affect tissue health and cell function. You can't feel it, but those tissues are hurting and inflamed. That inflammation needs to be significantly reduced or eliminated. That requires a special fatty acid.

You will also need to build, rebuild, and repair tissue. That requires a special fatty acid as well. The saturated fatty acids produced internally by the Brain-body System will do the job during fetal development and for other tissues, but the brain is special and requires a special fatty acid.

There are two unsaturated fatty acids that your brain needs; Omega-3 and Omega-6 fatty acids but they do different things. The primary difference is in their anti-inflammatory and clotting capabilities. Omega-3 has an anti-inflammatory capability. Omega-6 does not. Omega-6 helps with blood clotting Omega-3 does not. Omega-6 tends to be plentiful in the foods we eat whereas Omega-3 is scarce.

Omeg-3 polyunsaturated fatty acid is the fatty acid that your brain needs. It contains the acids e-p-a and d-h-a. E-p-a is an anti-inflammatory and d-h-a helps to repair and rebuild tissue. Omega-3 polyunsaturated fatty acid is an essential fatty acid because it can't be produced by the Brain-body System. It has to come from the foods you eat.

If you want a healthy brain it's important that you eat cold water fish, at least, twice a week. Add a green leafy salad while ingesting crushed flax seed and walnuts at other times. Flax seed works well on salads and in cereals. Build into its use gradually or your system will rebel. My suggestion is to start with one-half teaspoon a day and build gradually to one tablespoons a day. Check the appendix of this book for foods rich in Omega-3 polyunsaturated fatty acid.

If you like red meat in your diet you should know that unless you're eating free range, grass fed beef you're getting much more Omega-6 than is brain healthy. Too much Omega-6 will block the receptors for Omega-3 and result in some serious cell-damage. Omega-6 is needed, but is useful only in the right proportion to Omega-3. According to the World Health Organization that proportion should not exceed 10:1. Free range, grass fed beef has a ratio of about 2:1. Today's farmed, grain fed, beef has a ratio that approximates 23:1. If you are going to eat red meat make sure that it's free range and grass fed.

At this point you have a lot to think about and do with regard to your diet, but there is one more thing. Cholesterol and saturated fats are two fatty acids you don't have to ingest. You can't avoid them completely but you can minimize your intake. Saturated fatty acid and cholesterol are non-essential fatty acids produced internally. Your Brain-body System will produce all it needs using the foods you ingest. Excess amounts of saturated fat will be sent into the body as storage fat.

Cholesterol is a non-essential fatty acid. Your cells need cholesterol for structure, but your Brain-body system produces about 75% of all the cholesterol your cells need. The foods you consume provide the rest. Saturated fat does not contain any cholesterol, but the saturated fats that you consume will cause your system to produce cholesterol.

Cholesterol comes from animal products including dairy. Eating small amounts of foods containing cholesterol won't hurt, but if you like cheese, like I do, low-fat cheese probably won't work for you. Eat the good stuff just don't overdo. Eggs are great for providing protein and are cholesterol rich, but an average of one egg a day can be easily tolerated. It seems that the whole egg is better for you than just the egg whites.

If your diet contains more cholesterol than you need the excess will have nowhere to go. It gets deposited on your blood vessels and blocks blood flow limiting the oxygen, water and nutrients that your brain needs to function. That could have an effect on your cognitive abilities.

BACK TO LEARNING

Let's go back to processing new information, learning. "*Use it or lose it.*" You've heard it said often enough. The statement is obviously referring to older adults. They're probably out of their primary career, probably retired, and their younger children are telling them that they have to do something to keep their minds functioning. They push puzzles, games and mind stumpers on them. They mean well.

To start with, the statement should be "*Use it or lose it ... use it and improve it.*" Puzzles, games and mind stumpers are great for insight and mental agility, but other than the accomplishment of solving the puzzle or mind stumper the game has no significance. The mental logistics are the important part. There's no reason for you to remember the solution. That suggests that in most cases puzzles, games and mind stumpers don't really help build memory. When you process new information you should be learning.

To lead a brain healthy life style you should always be processing new information and learning something. Social interaction is a good way to process new information. Learn to do something that you've always wanted to do but never had the time or the opportunity to do. It makes no difference what you're learning as long as you're learning something. Combine social interaction with learning and you have a real winner. Good examples are classes dealing with a subject you would find interesting, group discussions and music lessons.

We live in the age of the internet which puts learning opportunities at your finger-tips. Unfortunately, it's a solitary experience, but if that's what you can do then do it. You need to be learning something. You can get your social interaction at other times in other ways. If you chose to go the route of the internet there are E-courses about almost everything. Check out your local library and see what they offer. You might be surprised at the CD and DVD, non-fiction, audio books that they offer. You just have to look for whatever turns you on.

Learning is not just for young children and young adults. Everyone needs to be learning something all the time regardless of age. Variations on what you already know don't count, but there are exceptions.

If you know how to use a computer learning a new and difficult computer program to do something that you've not done before would qualify as processing new information. If you play a musical instrument learning a new and challenging piece of music would qualify as processing new information. The three qualifiers are that it's new, different from what you already know, and it's stretching your abilities. To live a brain healthy life style you need to be learning and stretching your abilities, regardless of age. Your next step then is to search out and learn something new.

It seems that every time I mention this at a presentation someone in the audience will say "I work … I usually get home late … even when I get home early I'm tired … I want to relax … Learning something is the last thing I want to do … What am I supposed to do?"

That's a common and understandable situation. The first thing you need to accept is that continuing to learn is going to require persistence and effort. Learning doesn't mean that you have to be in a formal setting. It doesn't mean that you have to be learning something that stresses you out. Make it enjoyable. Pick something that you want to do.

I started to relearn the piano, something I've wanted to do for years. Take 15 minutes a day, in the morning, at lunchtime, during a break. What you do is up to you. All you need is 15 minutes a day, but you have to be consistent and repetitive in what you do. Just make sure that you do it. Give it time and your brain will respond.

STRESS AND SLEEP
Up to this point, to build a brain healthy life style you've dealt with the health of your sensors, your personal health, physical activity, hydration, the foods you eat and drink, and the processing of new information. There are two additional things left that need to be dealt with: stress and sleep. They can be considered polar opposites.

Stress is with us all the time. It's part of life. Stress is an anxiety that's brought about by what you need, what you're doing, and what might occur as a result of what you're doing. Stress is a survival response. Long term stress can be incredibly damaging to your cognitive plant.

You can't avoid stress, but you can manage it. How you manage it is up to you. Physical activity and exercise help, but there are two other things that I would like to suggest, and they're connected. Your brain has all kinds of things that constantly need attention, even when you sleep. Your brain never relaxes unless you give it the opportunity. Yet, your brain thrives if it does have some down time where it really doesn't have to do anything, where all of the emotional and environmental factors that its constantly dealing with are put into the background, suspended. This actually has a name. It's known as the relaxation response.

Given the opportunity to relax, your brain thrives coming back stronger than ever, particularly in the areas of focus and perspective. I'm talking about meditation. There is a related activity called "Mindful Awareness". Mindful Awareness helps you to focus on one thing at a time. Meditation blocks out everything and gives your brain a chance to relax.

You can meditate at any time doing almost anything. I meditate while working out on my hybrid treadmill-stairmaster. It's easy to do. You just have to learn what to do, but again everyone is a little different. What I do might not work for you, and what you do might not work for someone else. You have to find the right combination of elements that work for you. There are books, DVD's or you can consult a professional. There are a lot of inexpensive ways to get information about meditating and Mindful Awareness. You need to look into it.

The last thing that you need to deal with as part of a brain healthy life style is "*sleep*". Sleep is important because it's the brain's time to clean house administratively, and to repair and rebuild cells. Once into a brain healthy life style you should have no problem sleeping, but problems sleeping can be caused by physical or emotional factors.

The most common physical problem occurs when you've gotten into a sleep position that causes your hyoid bone to interfere with your breathing. If your hyoid bone interferes with your breathing the functioning of your heart and lungs will be affected causing blood flow to be slowed. The brain isn't getting what it needs and will wake you up. Emotional sleep problems can come from worry, anxiety, depression, stress, and lack of physical activity

If you've followed the path for a brain healthy life you should be sleeping well. If you're not than I would suggest that you review your life style to see what might be missing. I would also recommend seeing a doctor in case you have a physical problem.

SMOKING

There is one other thing, *smoking.* It appears that most people, smokers and non-smokers, understand the effects of smoking on the heart and lungs. They might pay more attention if they understood the effects of smoking on brain health and cognitive ability.

Smoking constricts blood vessels, reduces blood flow to the brain, and increases the possibility of a blood clot and stroke. When blood flow to the brain is decreased it has a direct impact on brain health and cell function, but it gets worse.

The smoke from cigarettes contains a variety of toxins including arsenic and cyanide. They get into the blood and circulate attacking cells and damaging cell function. Cells in the brain are particularly vulnerable to the toxins produced when smoking. Studies have shown that smoking causes a decline in cognitive ability, increases the risk of dementia and substantially increases the possibility of stroke as well as death from stroke.

If you want to lead a brain healthy life smoking is out.

Moving Into a Brain Healthy Life

I said it at the beginning of this section and I'll say it again. "You shouldn't feel that moving into a brain healthy life is a sacrifice that you're making to keep age from robbing you of your cognitive abilities. Quite the contrary. Moving into a brain healthy life style will open doors for you as you age that will take you into a new, exciting world.

Technology has not only changed the instruments that we have available to us, it's given us the information that we've needed, to know and understand our brain, to understand who we are. It's made us realize that our brain is all about the future and living. With that knowledge it's time that we removed ourselves from the past and moved into the future as we age. It's up to us and a healthy brain to do it.

"Your brain responds to what you do and don't do ... Determines what you can and can't do and decides what you will and won't do."

Appendix A

The Five Categories of Foods You

Need to Eat and Drink

1. Water

2. Anti-oxidants

3. Unsaturated Fat

4. Protein

5. Complex Carbohydrates

1. WATER

Hydration is essential to the functioning of the brain and Water is essential for hydration. Brain tissues and cells live in water. It's water that contains the foods that your brain feeds on. It's water that allows the cell enzymes to function. It's water that keeps the tissue and cells flexible. It's water that removes the waste and toxins, and its water that protects the brain from banging into that hard, bony, spiked thing that we refer to as a skull.

2. ANTI-OXIDANTS

Anti-oxidants are the brain's defense force. They defend against the onslaught of oxidants produced by the brain when converting fuel to energy. Glutathione is the brain's internally produced super anti-oxidant. The amount and types of foods we ingest today overwhelm the capabilities of glutathione. Glutathione has to be supported with foods rich in tyrosine, vitamins A, C and E. Tyrosine helps in the internal production of glutathione while foods rich in vitamins A, C and E are anti-oxidants that support the defensive behavior of glutathione.

Foods that support the production of Glutathione are:
asparagus, avocados, raw ripe green beans, red beets, kale, broccoli, Brussels sprouts, cabbage, onions, garlic, cauliflower, bok choy, watercress, mustard, horseradish, turnips, rutabagas, kohlrabi spices such as rosemary, tumeric, cinnamon, cardamom and cur cumin, whey protein powder, peaches, watermelon and Brazil nuts.

Foods rich in Vitamin E are:
broccoli, carrots, kale, grapes, onions, sweet potatoes, blueberries, spinach, oranges.

Foods rich in Vitamin A are
sweet potato (cooked), carrots (cooked), dark leafy greens (cooked) such as kale, spinach, collards, turnip greens, beet greens, Swiss chard, Pak Choi, romaine lettuce, green and red leaf lettuce, butterhead and chicory squash, butternut squash, pumpkin, and winter squash, cantaloupe melon, sweet red peppers, tropical fruits such as mango and papaya.

Foods rich in Vitamin C are:
apricots, beans. blackberries, cabbage, collard greens, chili peppers, gooseberries, grapefruit, lemon, lime, honeydew melon, okra, onion, oranges, prickly pears, radishes, raspberries, rutabaga, spinach, summer squash, tangerines, tomato, watermelon. papaya, bell peppers, broccoli,

Brussels sprout, strawberries, pineapple, oranges, kiwifruit, cantaloupe melon and cauliflower

FATTY ACIDS
All fats that are consumed enter the blood stream as fatty acids. There are two types of fatty acids.

> NON-ESSENTIAL FATS –Those that the body produces internally according to need. Non-Essential fats are saturated fat and cholesterol which is a steroidal fat.

> CHOLESTEROL – There are two different types of cholesterol; High Density Lipoprotein (HDL) and Low Density Lipoprotein (LDL). The term "Lipo" refers to a fatty acid. A Lipoprotein is a fatty acid combined with a protein. When doctors are talking to us about cholesterol they're talking about lipoproteins. LDL is a lipoprotein that has more fat than protein. HDL is a lipoprotein that has more protein than fat. Saturated fats do not contain cholesterol but ingesting foods containing saturated fat will cause the body to produce cholesterol.

> ESSENTIAL FATS – Those that the body CANNOT PRODUCE internally. Essential fats are monounsaturated and polyunsaturated fat. These fats must come directly from the foods you ingest.

3. UNSATURATED FATTY ACIDS
All unsaturated fatty acids are essential and are needed to build cell tissue. The brain can only use unsaturated fatty acids in the Omega-class. The fatty acids in the Omega class are Omega-3, Omega-6, Omega-7 and Omega-9 fatty acids. Omega-7 does not play a part in brain function. Omega-9 is a non-essential fatty acid that the Brain-body System produces when Omega-3 fatty acids aren't available. Omega-9 fatty acid is a very inefficient substitute for Omega-3 fatty acid.

Omega-6 Polyunsaturated Fatty Acid

Omega-6 fatty acid does not have an anti-inflammatory capability, which the brain needs, and will block the reception of Omega-3 when excessive quantities are present in the blood. Omega-6 fatty acid is prevalent in the foods we eat.

Foods rich in Omega-6 fatty acids are primarily Processed foods, fast foods, vegetable oils (e.g., corn, sunflower, safflower, soy and cottonseed oil), and farm raised, grain fed beef.

Omega-3 Polyunsaturated Fatty Acid

Omega-3 polyunsaturated fatty acid is important to brain health and brain function. The EPA component of Omega-3 fatty acid is an effective anti-inflammatory. It's DHA component provides the construction material the brain needs to repair and build tissue. The combination of the two components makes Omega-3 fatty acid a very important part of a brain-healthy diet.

Foods rich in Omega-3 fatty acids are Cold water fish such as, salmon, tuna, herring, cod, halibut, mackerel, trout, sardines, anchovies, ground flak seed, walnuts, almonds, green leafy veg-etables (lettuce, broccoli, kale, and spinach), legumes (kidney, navy, pinto and lima beans, and peas), citrus fruits, melons, and cherries..

4. PROTEIN

There are all kinds of protein in your brain. Different proteins do different things. Proteins are the workers. It's protein that makes things happen by building tissue, forming and energizing enzymes, and acting as neurotransmitters.

Neurotransmitters can energize and motivate you or frustrate and sedate you. They can make you sharp or slow you down. It's the brains neurotransmitters that allow cells to talk to each other tell-ing everyone in the network what needs to be done, what's been done, how you should react to what's been done, and what still needs doing. It's the neurotransmitters in your brain that signals when to take action regardless of whether that action is painting, walking, talking or calculating a problem in astrophysics. It's the signaling that takes place between cells that tells the enzymes when to go into action. Like neurotransmitters those enzymes are proteins. They're just different proteins. Without protein your brain cells couldn't talk to each other, and your brain function would slow down to a crawl.

A protein is comprised of amino acids. The formation of a "complete" protein requires nine "Essential" amino acids. "Essential" proteins are proteins that your System needs, but can't produce on its own. You have to eat foods that provide the nine "Essential" amino acids.

You can get all nine amino acids from foods derived from animals. Foods derived from plants contain amino acids as well, but there's a difference. Animals will provide all nine "Essential" amino acids forming a "complete" protein.

With the exception of Spirulina, a blue-green algae, the amino acid content of foods from plants is incomplete. You can't eat just one type of fruit or vegetable at a sitting and expect to get all nine "Essential" amino acids. Different foods derived from plants have different amino acid content.

When you consume a complete protein it's broken down and goes into your blood as amino acids. Your blood transports those amino acids to your brain where they're reassembled into the proteins that are needed. Once the amino acids are converted back into protein they know what job they have and can go to work when called on.

Like all workers, though, proteins get tired, deplete, and wear out over time. Unfortunately, your brain can't store amino acids It has to use the amino acids it receives to rebuild and replace its proteins on a real time basis. You need to have a diet that will provide a continuing source of "complete proteins".

Fish, red meat, poultry, eggs, yogurt and cheese are the animal foods rich in protein. Although processed animal meats such as sausage, ham, and bacon may have high protein counts, they also carry with them some serious health risks. Unless you're eating a low fat cheese it might be a good idea to look elsewhere for your protein. The same is true of yogurts. Although there's a lot of controversy surrounding eggs, it's agreed that they are great source of protein if you keep them down to an average of one per day.

Plant protein comes primarily from grains, legumes, seeds, nuts and fruit. Spirulina, a blue-algae, is the only plant food that seems to be rich in all nine essential amino acids. Other foods from plants, including fruit and some tubers like sweet potatoes, contain a complete compliment of amino acids, but may be weak in one or two. To be combined amino acids don't have to be consumed all together. An adult eating a varied, healthy diet based primarily on plant foods will receive a complete compliment of needed protein. However, infants and children have a greater need to digest a complete complement of all nine essential amino acids at the same meal.

5. CARBOHYDRATES

All carbohydrates are sugars. Carbohydrates are metabolized, and enter the blood as glucose. Glucose is the most efficient, energy producing fuel available to the Brain-body system.

Carbohydrates are typically sorted into two categories; simple carbohydrates and complex carbohydrates. Regardless of category, all carbohydrates are sugar. The sugars are converted into glucose and carried in your blood to where they're needed. Carbohydrates in both categories are potential sources of energy, but that's where the similarity stops.

Complex Carbohydrates ("Carbs")

Complex carbohydrates are the most efficient source of energy for the brain. Complex carbohydrates digest slowly due to their fiber content, they are a high powered, efficient source of energy, have significant nutrient value, and are low in fat. The foods richest in complex carbohydrates are whole grains, some seeds, fruit, vegetables and legumes.

Fiber

Complex carbohydrates contain fiber. Fiber is a structural component of plants, and has no nutrient value. Human digestive enzymes can't break it down allowing it to pass through the system without entering the blood. Because it passes through the system undigested it doesn't add calories to the diet. The fiber in foods slows the conversion of sugar to glucose allowing the glucose to enter the blood gradually. That helps to balance blood glucose levels minimizing the amount of toxic waste that has to be cleared by internal antioxidants.

Whole Grains

Whole grains are a good source of complex carbohydrates. They're high in fiber, rich in nutrients and low in fat. Whole grain or whole wheat refers to wheat that still contains the bran and germ. The bran is the covering that protects the germ, or embryo, of the wheat. It's rich in fiber, essential fatty acids, and contains protein, vitamins and minerals. The germ of the wheat is the most vitamin and mineral rich part of the wheat.

Examples of whole grains are wild rice, brown rice, oats, oat bran, cornmeal, barley, wheat germ, millet, buckwheat, and amaranth. Any foods made from these grains are a good source of complex carbs. Examples of whole grain products are breads, bagels, buns, rolls, pasta, macaroni, and whole grain breakfast cereals.

Fruit

Whole fruit is a complex carbohydrate. The juice of the fruit normally contains a good amount of sugar suggesting that fruit metabolizes and enters the blood quickly like a simple sugar. Whole fruit is typically high in fiber which slows the metabolic process allowing the sugar to enter your blood gradually. That makes whole fruit a good source of glucose and energy.

Whole fruit is also high in water content. Fruit skin and pulp contains anti-oxidants, vitamins, flavonoids and minerals. Whole fruit has little or no fat and is usually rich in protein. Tomatoes, squash, and cucumbers are categorized as fruit although they typically have less sugar than other types of whole fruit.

The skin and pulp inside are the healthy parts of the fruit and contain most of the fiber, minerals and vitamins. The pulpy part of fruit is the primary source of flavonoids. Flavonoids work in conjunction with the vitamins in the fruit to strengthen their health affect.

When making juice the skin, pulp and flavonoids are removed leaving just sugar. Commercially processed juice may say "pulp added", but the pulp may not be from the original fruit and is typically less than what was removed. In fruit juices flavonoids are lost completely.

Vegetables and Tubers

Vegetables and tubers have a good sugar content, typically contain a significant amount of water, and are low in fat. Like whole fruit vegetables and tubers are rich in anti-oxidants, vitamins and minerals. Artichokes, asparagus, broccoli, Brussels sprouts, cabbage, cauliflower, celery, carrots, corn, eggplant, lettuce of all types, onions potatoes, sweet potatoes, spinach, turnip greens, yams, and zucchini are all complex carbohydrates.

Legumes

Legumes are seeds that have a pod surrounding them, and are a good source of complex carbohydrates. Beans, such as kidney beans, black beans, garbanzo beans, soy beans, and pinto beans, lentils and peas are good examples of legumes.

Simple Carbohydrates

Simple carbohydrates don't normally have any nutrient or health value. They don't contain much, if any, fiber. Simple carbohydrates don't normally contain anti-oxidants, vitamins or minerals. Simple carbohydrates are typically sugar and non-essential fats.

When you ingest a simple carbohydrate there's nothing to slow down or regulate the amount of sugar going into the blood. All of the sugar is quickly converted to glucose and enters the blood in large amounts. The blood's sugar will increase to excessive levels (spike), possibly overwhelming the insulin response, and flooding the brain with glucose.

The brain can't store fuel. It can only productively use a limited amount of glucose at a time. If glucose arrives in the brain in excessive amounts it will be burned, but a considerable amount will be unused and wasted. More oxidants will be generated than can be neutralized and eliminated by the brain's internal defense force. That makes simple carbohydrates toxic to the brain and damaging to brain function.

Bibliography

Ordered By Date, Alphabetically By Author

2013

Kurzweil, Ray, (2013), How to Create a Mind, New York, NY, Penguin Books

David Perlmutter M.D. and Kristin Loberg, (2013), The Grain Brain: The Surprising Truth about Wheat, Carbs, and Sugar-Your Brain's Silent Killers, New York, NY, Little, Brown and Company

2012

Hyman, Mark M.D., (2012), Blood Sugar Solution: NY, New York, Little Brown & Co

2011

Cohen, Suzy R.Ph., (2011) Drug Muggers, New York, NY, Rodale, Inc.

Deacon, Terrence W., (2011) Incomplete Nature: How Mind Emerged From Matter, New York, W.W. Norton and Company Hoffecker, John F., (2011), Landscape of the Mind, New York, NY, Columbia University Press

David A., (2011), How the Brain Learns, Thousand Oaks, CA, Corwin Press

2010

Bowden, Jonny M.A., C.N.S., (2010), Living Low Carb: Controlled-Carbohydrate Eating for Long-Term, Trade Paperbacks

2009

Fields, R. Douglas PhD, (2009), The Other Brain, New York, NY, Simon & Schuster

Gordon, Dan, Editor, (2009), Cerebrum - Emerging Ideas in Brain Science: Washington, D.C., The Dana Press

Kessler, David A. M.D. (2009), The End of Overeating: NY, New York, Rodale, Inc.

Shealy, Norman C. M.D., PhD, (2009), Holy Water, Sacred Oil, The Fountain of Youth: Fair Grove, MO, Biogenics Books

Vernikos, Joan, PhD (2009), Stress Fitness for Seniors: Culpepper, VA, Thirdage llc.

2008

Amen, Daniel G. M.D., (2008), Magnificent Mind At Any Age, New York, NY, Random House, Inc.

Cozolino, Louis, (2008) The Healthy Aging Brain, New York, NY, W.W. Norton & Company

La Puma, John M.D., (2008), Chef MD's Big Book of Culinary Medicine: N.Y., New York, Crown Publishers

Ratey, John J. M.D., (2008), SPARK, New York, NY, Little Brown & Co.

La Puma, John M.D., (2008), Chef MD's Big Book of Culinary Medicine: N.Y., New York, Crown Publishers

2007

Begley, Sharon, (2007), Train Your Mind Change Your Brain. New York, NY, Ballantine

Bennett, Connie, C.H.H.C., (2007), Sugar Shock!: NY, New York, The Berkley Publishing Group

Bloom, Floyd E. M.D., (2007). Best of the Brain from Scientific American, Washington, D.C., The Dana Press

Bowden, Jonny PhD., C.N.S., (2007), Living the Low Carb Life", "150 healthiest Foods on Earth, Gloucester, MA, Quayside Publishing Group

Dodge, Norman M.D., (2007), the Brain that Changes Itself, Stories of Personal Triumph from the Frontiers of Brain Science, New York, NY, The Penguin Group.

Preuss, Harry M.D., Macn, CNS, and Gottlieb, Bill, (2007), The Natural Fat – Loss Pharmacy: N.Y., New York, Broadway Books

Prothero, Donald R. (2007), Evolution What the Fossils Say and Why It Matters: NY, New York, Columbia University Press

Taylor, Richard, (2007), Alzheimers from the Inside Out: Baltimore, MD, Health Professionals Press, Inc.

Sahelian, Ray M.D., (2007), Mind Boosting Secrets, Stamford, CT, Bottom Line Books

2006

Simon, Michael, (2006) "Appetite for Profit: How The Food Industry Undermines Our Health and How to Fight Back, New York, NY, Nation Books

Stewart, William B. M.D., (2006), Deep Medicine: Dexter, Michigan, Thomas-Shore, Inc.

2005

Bloom, Floyd E. M.D., (2005). Best of the Brain from Scientific American, Washington, D.C., The Dana Foundation

Noir, Michel PhD, and Croisile, Bernard M.D., PhD, (2005), Dental Floss for the Mind: New York, NY, McGraw Hill

Rose, Stephen, (2005), The Future of the Brain: The Promise and Perils of Tomorrows Neuroscience, New York, NY, Oxford University Press

Tan, Zaldy S. M.D., (2005), Age-Proof Your Mind: N.Y., New York, Warner Books

2004

Bransford, John D., Brown, Ann L., and Cocking, Rodney R., editors, (2004), How People Learn, Brain, Mind, Experience and School, Washington, D.C., National Academy Press

Norden, Jeanette PhD, (2004), Understanding the Brain, Chantilly, VA, The Great Courses

Shankle, Wm. Rodman M.S., M.D., and Amen, Daniel G. M.D., (2004), Preventing Alzheimer's, New York, NY, The Berkley Publishing Group

2003

Barnard, Neal M.D., (2003), Breaking the Food Seduction: N.Y., New York, St. Martin's Press

Batmanghelidj F. M.D., (2003), You're Not Sick You're Thirsty!: New York, NY, Warner Books

Batmanghelidj F. M.D., (2003), Water Cures: Drugs Kill, Vienna, VA, Global Health Solutions, Inc.

Bland, Jeffrey S. PhD, (2003), Improving Health Outcomes Through Nutritional Support for Metabolic Biotransformation, Seminar Series Syllabus: Gig Harbor, WA, Metagenics Educational Program

Poon, Leonard W. PhD, Gueldner, Sarah Hall DSN, FAAN, Sprouse, Betsy M PhD., Editors, (2003), Successful Aging and Adaption with Chronic Diseases, New York, NY, Springer Publishing

Speight, Neal, M.D., Program Chairperson, (2003) Genetic and Environmental Influences on the Nervous System: Los Vegas, American College for Advancement in Medicine

2002

Begley, Sharon, (2002), The Mind and the Brain: Neuroplasticity and the Power of Mental Force, New York, NY, HarperCollins Publishers

Schwartz, Jeffrey M., (2002), The Mind and The Brain, New York, NY, HarperCollins Publishers

2001

McFadden, John Joe, (2001), Quantum Evolution, New York, NY, W.W. Norton & Company

Ratey, John M.D., (2001), A User's Guide to the Brain, New York, Pantheon Books

Wade, Nicholas, Editor, (2001), Book of the Brain, Guilford, Connecticut, The Lyons Press

1999

Editors of Scientific American, (1999), The Brain: Guilford, Connecticut, The Globe Pequot Press

Roizen, Michael F. M.D., (1999), Real Age, Are You as Young as You Can Be?: New York, NY, HarperCollins Publishers, Inc.

VanderHaeghe, Lorna, and Bouic. J.D. PhD (1999) The Immune System Cure: New York, New York, Kensington Books

1998

Dowling, John E.. (1998), Creating Mind, New York, NY, W.W. Norton & Company

Wade, Nicholas, Editor, (1998), Articles, Book of the Brain, New York Times, Guilford, CT, the Lyons Press

1997

Deacon, Terrence W., (1997), The Symbolic Species, New York, NY, W.W. Norton & Company

Lombard, Jay M.D., and Germano, Carl RD, CNS, LDN, (1997), The Brain Wellness Plan, New York, NY, Kensington Publishing Company

Mayr, Ernst, (1997), This is Biology, Cambridge, MA, The Belknap Press of Harvard University Press

Pinker, Steven, (1997), How the Mind Works, New York, W.W. Norton & Company

1995

Gatz, M. (1995). Emerging issues in mental health and aging. Washington, DC: American Psychological Association.

Weil, Andrew M.D., (1995), Spontaneous Healing: NY, New York, Alfred A. Knopf

1994

Black, Ira B., (1994), Information in the Brain: Cambridge, MA, The MIT Press

Thomas, John, (1994), Young Again!, Keiso, Washington, Plexus Press

1992

Batmanghelidj F. M.D., (1992), Your Body's Many Cries for Water: New York, NY, GHS, Inc.

1991

Black, Ira B., (1991), Information on the Brain, A Molecular Perspective, Cambridge, MA, Bradford Books

Restak, Richard M.D., (1991), The Brain Has a Mind of its Own: Insights From a Practicing Neurologist, New York, NY, Crown Publications

1990

Chopra, Deepak, (1990), Quantum Healing, New York, Bantam Books

Norton S. Beckerman

Prior to 1990, alphabetically by author

Benson, Herbert M.D., (1975), The Relaxation Response, New York, NY, Harper Collins Publishers, Inc.

Ford, E.B., (1979), Understanding Genetics, New York, NY, Pica Press

Hanson, Peter G. M.D., (1985), The Joy of Stress: Kansas City, MO, McMeel & Parker Universal Press

Krupp, E.C. PhD, (1983), Echoes of the Ancient Skies, New York, NY, Harper & Row

Minderhoud, J.M., Editor, (1981), Cerebral Blood Flow, Basic Knowledge and Clinical Implications: Netherlands, Antilles, Excerpta Medica

Moyers, Bill, (1979), Healing and the Mind, New York, NY, Doubleday

Oakley, David A., Editor (1985), Brain & Mind: New York, NY, Methuen, Inc.

Ornstein, Robert PhD and Sobel, David M.D., (1989), Healthy Pleasures: Reading Massachusetts, Perseus Books

Reneman, R.S., Maastricht, Bollinger, A., and Zurich, volume editors, (1985), Serotonin and microcirculation: Proceedings of Symposium at the Third World Congress for Microcirculation: Basel. Switzerland, Karger, A.G.

Smith, Bernard H. M.D., (1979), Differential Diagnosis in Neurobiology: New York, New York, Arco Publishing

Solomon, Eldra Pearl and Davis P. William, (1983), Human Anatomy and Physiology: Japan, McGraw-Hill, Inc.

Thomas, Lewis, (1974), The Lives of a Cell: New York, NY, Viking Penguin Press

Yankelovich, Daniel (1981), New Rules: New York, NY, Random House, Inc.

Bibliography

Alphabetically By Author's Last Name

A

Amen, Daniel G. M.D., (2008), Magnificent Mind At Any Age, New York, NY, Random House, Inc.

B

Barnard, Neal M.D., (2003), Breaking the Food Seduction: N.Y., New York, St. Martin's Press

Batmanghelidj F. M.D., (2003), You're Not Sick You're Thirsty!: New York, NY, Warner Books

Batmanghelidj F. M.D., (2003), Water Cures: Drugs Kill, Vienna, VA, Global Health Solutions, Inc.

Batmanghelidj F. M.D., (1992), Your Body's Many Cries for Water: New York, NY, GHS, Inc.

Bennett, Connie, C.H.H.C., (2007), Sugar Shock!: NY, New York, The Berkley Publishing Group

Benson, Herbert M.D., (1975), The Relaxation Response, New York, NY, Harper Collins Publishers, Inc.

Black, Ira B., (1994), Information in the Brain: Cambridge, MA, The MIT Press

Black, Ira B., (1991), Information in the Brain, Cambridge, MA, The MIT Press

Bland, Jeffrey S. PhD, (2003), Improving Health Outcomes Through Nutritional Support for Metobolic Biotransformation, Seminar Series Syllabus: Gig Harbor, WA, Metagenics Educational Program

Bloom, Floyd E. M.D., Editor, (2007). Best of the Brain from Scientific American, Washington, D.C., The Dana Press

Bloom, Floyd E. M.D., Editor, (2005). Best of the Brain from Scientific American, Washington, D.C., The Dana Foundation

C

Cohen, Suzy RPh, (2011) Drug Muggers, New York, NY, Rodale, Inc.

E

Editors of Scientific American, (1999), The Brain: Guilford, Connecticut, The Globe Pequot Press

F

Fields, R. Douglas PhD, (2009) The Other Brain, New York, NY, Simon & Schuster

Ford, E.B., (1979), Understanding Genetics, New York, NY, Pica Press

G

Gordon, Dan, Editor, (2009), Cerebrum - Emerging Ideas in Brain Science: Washington, D.C., The Dana Press

H

Hanson, Peter G. M.D., (1985), The Joy of Stress: Kansas City, MO, McMeel & Parker Universal Press

Hoffecker, John F., (2011), Landscape of the Mind, New York, NY, Columbia University Press

Hyman, Mark M.D., (2012), Blood Sugar Solution: NY, New York, Little Brown & Co

K

Kessler, David A. M.D. (2009), The End of Overeating: NY, New York, Rodale, Inc.

Krupp, E.C. PhD, (1983), Echoes of the Ancient Skies, New York, NY, Harper & Row

Kurzweil, Ray, (2013), How to Create a Mind, New York, NY, Penguin Books

L

La Puma, John M.D., (2008), Chef MD's Big Book of Culinary Medicine: N.Y., New York, Crown Publishers

Le Doux, Joseph. (1996), The Emotional Brain, New York, NY., Touchstone Press

Le Doux, Joseph. (2003), The Synaptic Self: How Our Brain Becomes Who We are, New York, NY., Penguin Press

Lombard, Jay M.D., and Germano, Carl RD, CNS, LDN, (1997), The Brain Wellness Plan, New York, NY, Kensington Publishing Company

M

Mayr, Ernst, (1997), This is Biology, Cambridge, MA, The Belknap Press of Harvard University Press

McFadden, John Joe, (2001), Quantum Evolution, New York, NY, W.W. Norton & Company

Minderhoud, J.M., Editor, (1981), Cerebral Blood Flow, Basic Knowledge and Clinical Implications: Netherlands, Antilles, Excerpta Medica

Moyers, Bill, (1979), Healing and the Mind, New York, NY, Doubleday

N

Noir, Michel PhD, and Croisile, Bernard M.D., PhD, (2005), Dental Floss for the Mind: New York, NY, McGraw Hill

Norden, Jeanette PhD, (2004), Understanding the Brain, Chantilly, VA, The Great Courses

O

Oakley, David A., Editor (1985), Brain & Mind: New York, NY, Methuen, Inc.

Ornstein, Robert PhD and Sobel, David M.D., (1989), Healthy Pleasures: Reading Massachusetts, Perseus Books

P

Poon, Leonard W. PhD, Gueldner, Sarah Hall DSN, FAAN, Sprouse, Betsy M PhD., Editors, (2003), Successful Aging and Adaption with Chronic Diseases, New York, NY, Springer Publishing

Preuss, Harry M.D., Macn, CNS, and Gottlieb, Bill, (2007), The Natural Fat – Loss Pharmacy: N.Y., New York, Broadway Books

Prothero, Donald R. (2007), Evolution What the Fossils Say and Why It Matters: NY, New York, Columbia University Press

R

Ratey, John J. M.D., (2008), SPARK, New York, NY, Little Brown & Co.

La Puma, John M.D., (2008), Chef MD's Big Book of Culinary Medicine: N.Y., New York, Crown Publishers

Reneman, R.S., Maastricht, Bollinger, A., and Zurich, volume editors, (1985), Serotonin and microcirculation: Proceedings of Symposium at the Third World Congress for Microcirculation: Basel. Switzerland, Karger, A.G.

Roizen, Michael F. M.D., (1999), Real Age, Are You as Young as You Can Be?: New York, NY, HarperCollins Publishers, Inc.

S

Sahelian, Ray M.D., (2007), Mind Boosting Secrets, Stamford, CT, Bottom Line Books

Shealy, Norman C. M.D., PhD, (2009), Holy Water, Sacred Oil, The Fountain of Youth: Fair Grove, MO, Biogenics Books

Shankle, Wm. Rodman M.S., M.D., and Amen, Daniel G. M.D., (2004), Preventing Alzheimer's, New York, NY, The Berkley Publishing Group

Sinatra, Steven M.D., Bennett, Connie, C.H.H.C., (2007), Sugar Shock!: NY, New York, The Berkley Publishing Group

Smith, Bernard H. M.D., (1979), Differential Diagnosis in Neurobiology: New York, New York, Arco Publishing

Solomon, Eldra Pearl and Davis P.William, (1983), Human Anatomy and Physiology: Japan, McGraw-Hill, Inc.

Sousa, David A., (2011), How The Brain Learns, Thousand Oaks, CA, Corwin Press

Stewart, William B. M.D., (2006), Deep Medicine: Dexter, Michigan, Thomas-Shore, Inc.

Speight, Neal, M.D., Program Chairperson, (2003) Genetic and Environmental Influences on the Nervous System: Los Vegas, American College for Advancement in Medicine

T

Tan, Zaldy S. M.D., (2005), Age-Proof Your Mind: N.Y., New York, Warner Books

Taylor, Richard, (2007), Alzheimers from the Inside Out: Baltimore, MD, Health Professionals Press, Inc.

Thomas, John, (1994), Young Again!, Keiso, Washington, Plexus Press

Thomas, Lewis, (1974), The Lives of a Cell: New York, NY, Viking Penguin Press

V

VanderHaeghe, Lorna, and Bouic. J.D. PhD (1999) The Immune System Cure: New York, New York, Kensington Books

Vernikos, Joan, PhD (2009), Stress Fitness for Seniors: Culpepper, VA, Thirdage llc.

W

Wade, Nicholas, Editor, (2001), Book of the Brain, Guilford, Connecticut, The Lyons Press

Weil, Andrew M.D., (1995), Spontaneous Healing: NY, New York, Alfred A. Knopf

Y

Yankelovich, Daniel (1981), New Rules: New York, NY, Random House, Inc.

Bibliography

Publications and Internet Sources

Erickson, K., Exercise Training Increases Size of Hippocampus and Improves Memory, Proceedings of the National Academy of Sciences, published online (January 31, 2011)

Zimmer, Carl, 100 Trillion Connections, Scientific American, (January, 2011),

Marean, Curtis W., When the Sea Saved Humanity, Scientific American, (August, 2010).

Pritchard, Jonathan K., How We Are Evolving, Scientific American, (October 2010).

Zilhao, Joao, Did Neanderthals Think Like Us?, Scientific American, (June, 2010).

Pollard, Katherine B., What Makes Us Human?, Scientific American, (May, 2009).

Sanders, Laura, Exercise Helps Brains Bounce Back, Science News, Vol. 176, (November 21, 2009), p.8

Society for Neuroscience Annual Meeting, Chicago, IL, Junk Food Turns Rats Into Addicts, (October 17, 2009).

Technology Review, Time Travel Through the Brain, (November-December, 2009).

Berns, Gregory, Rewiring the Creative Mind, Fast Company, (October, 2008).

John Hopkins Medical Letter, Health After 50, Blood Pressure's Link to Dementia,, (December, 2006).

Amen, Daniel M.D., (December 31, 2002), Optimizing Brain Function, Brain & Mind Magazine, retrieved from:

http://www.cerebromente.org.br/n16/opiniao/seven-ways3.htm

Caine, Geoffrey and Renate Nummela, What "Whole Brain Means: Why Wholeness Matters", New Horizons, (September, 24, 2010), retrieved from: http://www.newhorizons.org/neuro/caine_whole.htm

Harvard School of Public Health, (March 14, 2011) the Nutrition Source, Fats and Cholesterol: Out with the bad, in with the good, retrieved from:

http://www.hsph,harvard.edu/nutritionsource/whatshouldyoueat/fatsandcholesterol

Russell, W. Ritchie, M.D., The Brain, A Journal of Neurobiology, Oxford Journals, Medicine, Brain, 132, Issue 3, pp. 565-567, Cerebral involvement in Head Injury. Retrieved from: http://brain.oxfordjournals.org/content/132/3/565

How (Brain) Cells Communicate, Prof Mark Girolami, Prof Miles Houslay and Prof Graeme Milligan; Prof Walter Kolch, www.PhysOrg.com

Internet Sources

PubMed Health http://ww.nebi.nlm.nikh.gov/pubmedhealth/
PMHOOO4546

Journal of Pediatric Psychiatry http://jpepsy.oxfordyournals.org/
content/22/1/59.short

Keith L. Black, M.D. and Cedars-Sinai: www.everydayhealth.com/
conditions/brain-nerves

www.MyBrainTunnels.com

www.aarp.org/health/brainhealth

www.alz.org

www.brainready.com/blog/thetop5brainhealthfoods.html

www.amenclinics.com

www.aarpmagazine.org/health/boost-brain-health.html

www.cerebralhealth.com

www.GoVeg.com/alzheimers.asp

www.my.clevelandclinic.org/brain_health/default.aspx

www.usnews.com/health-conditions/brain-health

www.fitbrains.com/science/health.usnews.com/brain-health.html

www.toptenz.net/top-10-foods-for-brain-health.php

www.keepmemoryalive.org/Pages/aspx

www.centerforbrainhealth.net/

www.brainhealth.com

www.BrainTumorTreatment.com

http://sites.lafayette.edu/neur401-sp10/researcher-profiles/elizabeth-gould/

http://brain-health-neurology.factoidz.com/is-memory-loss-just-a-sad-reality-of-aging/

http://bjp.rcpsycg.orgg/cgi/pdf_extract/42/179/744Neuroplasticity_is_not_a_new_discovery

---

www.ingramcontent.com/pod-product-compliance
Lightning Source LLC
Chambersburg PA
CBHW060306290526
45789CB00001B/416